Necessary S...

Necessary Scars
A Doctor's Life in Error

Philip Berry MBChB, MD, FRCP

Consultant Physician and Gastroenterologist,
St Thomas Hospital, London, UK

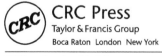

CRC Press

Taylor & Francis Group

Boca Raton London New York

CRC Press is an imprint of the
Taylor & Francis Group, an **informa** business

First edition published 2022
by CRC Press
6000 Broken Sound Parkway NW, Suite 300, Boca Raton, FL 33487-2742
and by CRC Press
2 Park Square, Milton Park, Abingdon, Oxon, OX14 4RN

© 2022 Taylor & Francis Group, LLC

CRC Press is an imprint of Taylor & Francis Group, LLC

Library of Congress Cataloging–in–Publication Data
Names: Berry, Philip (Consultant physician and gastroenterologist), author.
Title: Necessary scars : a doctor's life in error / Philip Berry.
Description: First edition. I Boca Raton : CRC Press, 2021. I Includes bibliographical references and index. I Summary: "The stories and discussions in the book provide detailed narratives, analyses and reflections on medical errors through actions, omissions and misunderstandings. They offer a unique perspective on the social implications of medical error and enable healthcare workers at all levels to analyse & learn from it"-- Provided by publisher.
Identifiers: LCCN 2021031254 (print) I LCCN 2021031255 (ebook) I ISBN 9781032039398 (hardback) I ISBN 9781032039374 (paperback) I ISBN 9781003189824 (ebook)
Subjects: MESH: Medical Errors I Personnel, Hospital--psychology I Personal Narrative
Classification: LCC R729.8 (print) I LCC R729.8 (ebook) I NLM WX 153 I DDC 610.289--dc23
LC record available at https://lccn.loc.gov/2021031254
LC ebook record available at https://lccn.loc.gov/2021031255

ISBN: 978-1-032-03939-8 (hbk)
ISBN: 978-1-032-03937-4 (pbk)
ISBN: 978-1-003-18982-4 (ebk)

DOI: 10.1201/9781003189824

Typeset in Times
by MPS Limited, Dehradun

Contents

Acknowledgements vii
Introduction ix
General Notes: Confidentiality xiii
Glossary xv

1   Deeds: Mistaken Actions and Reactions 1
    1.1   Flying 1
    1.2   Slick 2
    1.3   Shock 3
    1.4   Pride 5
    1.5   Listen 8
    1.6   Patterns 10
    1.7   Ignorant 14
    1.8   Stop 16
    1.9   Wait 17
    1.10 Trust 18
    1.11 Paralysis 19
    1.12 Zone 23
    1.13 Prison 24
    1.14 Burn 27

2   Words: Failures in Communication 31
    2.1   Limit 31
    2.2   Proximity 32
    2.3   Radius 33
    2.4   Comfort 34
    2.5   Cruel 35
    2.6   Loose 39
    2.7   Signals 40
    2.8   Privacy 42
    2.9   Unwanted 43
    2.10 Low 45
    2.11 Edge 46
    2.12 Dance 47

3   Skin: Resilience **51**
   3.1   Right 51
   3.2   Wall 53
   3.3   Stick 54
   3.4   Distance 55
   3.5   Sweat 65
   3.6   Guilt 68
   3.7   Sorry 70
   3.8   Poison 76
   3.9   Try 78
   3.10   Burst 79
   3.11   Curve 83
   3.12   Judgement 87
   3.13   Fear 90
   3.14   Eyeroll 94

4   Infamy: On Judgement and Punishment **103**
   4.1   Cross 103
   4.2   Peer 105
   4.3   Jack 108
   4.4   Maw 112
   4.5   Whistle 116
   4.6   Tunnel 124
   4.7   Rainstorm 127

Summing Up **133**

Endnotes **135**

Index **139**

Acknowledgements

'Paralysis' first appeared as 'Action v inaction: a case history in ethics' in *Journal of Medical Ethics*, 2003 Aug;29(4):225–6. Published with permission.

A section of 'Wall' first appeared in 'The Gut Thump' in *The Lancet* (24 June 2000).

Introduction

Friday afternoon in the hospital. Emma, a junior doctor qualified for almost a year, stands over the bed of an elderly patient called Lily Reeves. Lily was admitted to hospital with a stroke two weeks earlier, but her temperature has now dropped to 35.2°C – an ominous sign. Elderly patients do not always mount a fever to infection; sometimes their immune systems do not have the energy to put up a fight and they just succumb.

Emma diagnoses a urine infection and prescribes an antibiotic that is injected directly into the vein, trusting that it will get to work faster than tablets. But she fails to check the result of a urine sample that was taken three days before, when Lily first described some stinging.

The bacterial species causing the infection was isolated, cultured and tested against all the common antibiotics: it is resistant to the antibiotic that Emma chooses. During Friday night and Saturday morning, the bacteria multiply and spread into Lily's blood, leading to septicaemia. She shows no interest in breakfast on Sunday morning and descends rapidly into septic shock by lunchtime. At the age of 92, with known heart disease, a recent stroke and moderately advanced dementia, she is deemed too frail to benefit from transfer to the intensive care unit (ICU). All the ward nurses and the weekend doctors can do is call Lily's family in and keep her comfortable. Lily dies in the early hours of Monday morning.

At 8.30 AM, Emma enters the ward and immediately asks where the elderly lady in bed 18 has gone. Another junior doctor tells her what happened and mentions that it turned out Lily was receiving the 'wrong' antibiotic. Emma is devastated. She understands her error. The floor tilts beneath her feet. Her breathing becomes rapid and shallow.

Later, Emma's educational supervisor calls her in for 'a word'. He has received an email from one of the weekend team describing Lily's death and the incorrect prescription. There is no punishment, only an appeal that Emma 'reflects' on the error.

For days and weeks, Emma broods on her mistake. It is punishment enough. Vivid images of Lily and her family keep intruding on Emma's mind. For a fortnight, she wishes she had never studied medicine at all. There must be easier jobs, with less risk and less responsibility. She is thankful that her consultant protects her from the family when they attend the ward for a meeting, but she hears all about it.

'How could a simple urine infection go this far?' Lily's son asked in the meeting. Emma's consultant explained that bacteria in the bladder and kidneys can cause serious illness. These infections are never trivial. He also admits that a culture and sensitivity result went unheeded, and that the hospital is conducting an internal investigation into the matter.

Emma fears that it will go down on her record, but there is no such thing. Her supervisor mentions it in an end-of-placement review, but it is not a serious enough error to impede her progress or destroy her career.

'We've all done it,' he says.

In August, Emma moves on to a new job in a different hospital. Now she supervises two doctors who are junior to her (newly qualified staff are perpetually falling off the end of the medical school conveyor belt). Emma annoys them because she is such a stickler for detail. She clearly does not trust them – she is always checking the computer for results, and on every ward round asks, 'Are there any cultures? Have you checked the resistance profile?' The two lads (they happen to be male doctors, tanned after a final summer of freedom in the surf, who roam the ward seemingly without a care in the world) have no idea what happened to Emma, nor to Lily Reeves. But they learn Emma's ways and keep the results file up to date.

Emma carries that reputation for precision and double-checking with her throughout her training.

Twelve years later, now a fully trained respiratory specialist, Emma is asked to deliver an induction lecture to a room full of newly qualified doctors. She emphasises how important it is to take nothing for granted ... to watch the *details*. It is the details that matter, she explains; it is the details that kill.

She drives home at the end of the day and casts her mind back to the moment she learned that her elderly patient had died, due, in part, to her oversight. Strangely, she cannot remember the lady's name. She cannot recreate her face in her mind's eye. And the family ... how many were there? A son, was it? It is history now. Only the lesson that grew out of that error remains. The memory of Lily Reeves has been subsumed in Emma's memory by a decade of experience, by thousands of other patients, and by hundreds of other lessons.

In one of Martin Scorsese's least successful films, *Bringing Out The Dead* (1999),[1] a burned-out paramedic Frank Pierce sees the spectral forms of patients he failed to save rise through the sidewalks to torment him. When I saw this, I thought it was overly romantic. Later, I read a Tweet from a doctor: *'Whenever I have a couple of drinks, I think of all my patients who have passed away, even years before'.* What?! Really? I wondered if I had a circuit missing. Was I incapable of feeling? Surely, I asked myself, we cannot be expected to remember every patient who has died under our care. In the same way, I do not remember the name of every patient who may have suffered through an error I made. Perhaps that sounds heartless, but it is true. Later, I came to realise it is acceptable to process suffering and medical misfortune in your own way, be that with overt displays of feeling or a brief pang of regret on the corridor, as long as you learn something from it and use it to become a better doctor. The duty is not to feel everything, but to become better.

Mistakes are inevitable. The consequences of those mistakes are seared into our memories, and when we approach a similar set of circumstances months, years or decades later, we feel the scar rising from the surface of a familiar landscape and change direction.

The lifelong process of learning in a medical career requires us to find a way to live through these setbacks and make something positive out of them. To do this, doctors must strip those memories of the very qualities that made them so powerful in the first place ... the patients' suffering and the impact on their families or loved ones. The lesson learnt may be about data interpretation, practical technique or communication, or it may be about process or organisational structure. Whatever it is it is, the doctor must be involved in trying to reveal the cause. This requires objectivity. It is the emotion of the incident that causes the wound, but the healing will depend on the cool salve of analysis. The scar that remains must be visible, but it should not hurt any more. There are many more patients to be seen, and they cannot be served through a persistent fog of regret.

While objectivity is necessary, it must wait its turn. If we become too good at the process of assimilation and are tempted to put mistakes 'down to experience' too soon, there is a risk that we will not dwell sufficiently on the human impact of our mistakes. If we smoothly compartmentalise those errors, surrounding (or hiding) them in hastily erected walls of rationalisation, forensic examination and (instinctive) defensiveness, we may underplay their social significance. But if we *feel* each mistake at a deep emotional level for too long, we may burn out and leave medicine for good. There is a balance. We should not develop too thick a skin, but we must not be rendered weak through a thousand cuts. It was to help myself and others find that balance that I wrote this book.

The only doctor we can observe over an entire career is the one we see in the mirror every morning. This book recounts many of my own mistakes, and a few that I saw happen around me. The associated scars pepper the landscape of my mind and serve as warnings. Whether you are a doctor, a student or an otherwise interested reader, they may help you to understand how medicine works.

General Notes
Confidentiality

The popularity of medical memoirs has meant thousands of real patient stories now exist in print, and I am sure very few of those individuals gave written or verbal permission.[2] The way around this is to anonymise cases, to change or omit age and gender, and to erase as many specifics as possible. In that way, the chance of a patient (or a patient's relative) reading about themselves and recognising their own story is minimised. The events described in this book occurred over a 25-year period and contain no identifiable information. The dialogue is paraphrased. I cannot remember the names of the patients involved (as I admitted, via the voice of Emma, in the introduction). If each episode comes across as entirely believable, that is good. It means the essence of the case has been successfully transmitted to the reader. But the likelihood of the original patient being identified is negligible.

For example, in 'Pride', I write: *'Years later, working on an ICU, I admitted a young female patient with liver failure called Maghadi Padam.'*

The name is made up. I saw tens, perhaps hundreds, of patients with that life-threatening diagnosis. It would be impossible for even the most inquisitive reader to trace the patient who inspired this chapter. But a name is necessary; it completes the image for the reader.

How have other authors addressed this issue? Kathryn Mannix, in her marvellous book *With The End in Mind* (William Collins, 2018), writes:

> This is a book about real events. Everything described really happened to someone, sometime, in the last 40 years. To preserve the anonymity of the people described, almost all names have been changed, along with their jobs, and sometimes their gender or ethnicity. Because these are stories rather than case histories, sometimes the experience of several people is woven into a single individual narrative, to allow specific aspects of the journey to be depicted.

Fact and fiction merge, in this kind of writing, allowing the authors to communicate the kernel of truth. In *Necessary Scars,* I have changed many details, but I have not pieced different stories together. I have also been explicit when cases or dialogues are entirely made up; indeed, some scenarios have alternative endings (for example, 'Burn' and 'Curve'). I am also a fiction writer, and that may show through now and again. But this book is based in truth.

In my view, the benefit of sharing medical stories outweighs the very small risk of self-identification, if those stories are told sensitively and responsibly. The future of medicine depends on individuals passing on their learning. Without stories of success and failure, medicine would not have moved on from the days of blood-letting and heavenly invocation.

The COVID-19 Pandemic

Since starting this book, healthcare workers around the world have experienced something that they probably had not imagined would happen during their lifetime — a lethal pandemic. Any book that seeks to explore psychological scars inflicted at work must acknowledge its impact. Many young or inexperienced doctors and nurses will have seen more suffering during 2020–21 than they would otherwise have witnessed over a whole career. The consequences of this exposure remain to be seen. This book is about our involvement in error and harm, rather than our proximity to natural death. I will leave that subject to future authors.

Medical Terms

Although intended primarily for those contemplating, studying for or already in the healthcare profession, I hope this book will interest a general readership. Medical and scientific terms are explained in the main text, in footnotes and in a glossary.

NOTES

1. Based on a book by Joe Connelly, it bombed, making $16.8 million in receipts against $32 million production costs. Speaking to Roger Ebert, a film critic who adored the film, Scorsese said 'I had 10 years of ambulances. My parents, in and out of hospitals. Calls in the middle of the night. I was exorcising all of that. Those city paramedics are heroes—and saints, they're saints. I grew up next to the Bowery, watching the people who worked there, the Salvation Army, Dorothy Day's Catholic Worker movement, all helping the lost souls. They're the same sort of people.' (*Howard's end: Scorsese and 'The Aviator'*: RogerEbert.com 12.12.2004)

2. Matt Morgan, the author of *Critical: Science and Stories from the Brink of Human Life* (Simon & Schuster, 2019), is one of the exceptions. He has made it very clear that permission was given from each of the patients (or their family) described in his book. Writing in the *British Medical Journal* (*BMJ*, 5.12.2019) he explained 'All the people I visited wanted their story to be told and some even insisted on using their real names in the book. This was a surprise to me and the publishers. The ways to navigate this territory are unclear—I hope the approach that I took put patients firmly at the centre of concerns rather than the book. Using stories only where consent was possible did restrict those that I could include, but this was a price worth paying for maintaining trust.'

Glossary

Adrenaline: a powerful inotrope, a drug that strengthens cardiac function

Anecdote: when used in a medical context, this suggests a one-off observation that although compelling or memorable, should not have undue influence on future practice or decisions

Aspirin: simple pain killer which also thins the blood and helps reduce blood clotting in heart attacks

Balloon pump: a device with a narrow balloon that when inserted into the main blood vessel coming from the heart increases blood pressure and blood flow

Cannula: small plastic tube inserted into a vein through which drugs can be injected

Cardiologist: heart specialist

Contraindication: a reason not to give a particular treatment

CPAP (continuous positive airway pressure): a tight face mask that allows air to be pushed into the lungs under pressure, causing the lungs to inflate more effectively

Defibrillation:restoration of a regular electrical rhythm in the heart by administering an large electric shock

Diabetic retinopathy: disease of the retina, at the back of the eye, due to diabetes

Diuretic: a drug that stimulates the kidney and causes the patient to pass a lot of urine

Dobutamine: an inotrope, a drug that strengthens cardiac function

Echocardiogram: ultrasound of the heart, showing how the heart muscle and heart valves are working

External jugular vein: large vein in the neck, which if swollen and distended indicates heart failure

Infarcted: death of any part of the body (usually heart muscle) due to a blocked artery

Inotropes: a drug that increases the power of the heart

Haemofiltration: similar to dialysis, allowing the blood to be cleaned of the toxins that the kidneys would usually filter out

Hypoxic: low oxygen levels

Interventricular septum: membrane that separates the main chambers of the heart

Joules: measure of electric current

Mitral valve: one of four heart valves, integral to adequate heart function

Morphine: a powerful injected pain killer; can cause drowsiness and slow down breathing

Murmur: a humming sound in the heart heard with a stethoscope, caused by turbulent blood flow through abnormal valves or a hole in the heart

Naloxone: antidote to opiates (e.g., morphine, heroine)

PEEP: positive end expiratory pressure, a measurement used in mechanical ventilation

Pericardiocentesis: insertion of a needle into the membranous sac around the heart to drain a dangerous build of fluid

Pneumothorax/pneumothoraces: the edge of the lung is punctured (in an accident, or if the lung tissue is weakened by infection, cancer or degeneration), allowing air to leak into the space between the lung and the ribcage; if too much gas accumulates the lung collapses, and pressure can build up on the heart causing death

Precordial: the part of the chest in front of the heart

Pulmonary oedema: a build of fluid in the lungs

Strongyloides: parasite, a type of very small worm that can invade and multiply in many tissues, especially if the patient's immune system is weak.

Tamponade: dangerous compression of the heart due to build of fluid within the pericardial sac; the fluid can stop the heart pumping altogether

Thrombolyse: dissolving a blood clot

VF (ventricular fibrillation): rapid, chaotic heart electrical rhythm, resulting in inability of heart to pump

VSD (ventriculoseptal defect): a hole in the membrane separating the main chambers of the heart

1

Deeds: Mistaken Actions and Reactions

1.1 Flying

When everything goes well, medicine is immensely satisfying. When years of learning culminate in a correct diagnosis, when months of training result in a perfectly executed operation or procedure and when the patient improves, avoiding death or permanent disability, the doctor can walk away full of pride. This emotional journey, starting in the foothills of uncertainty and doubt, rising through self-validation, confirmation and, maybe, a moment of glory at the summit, is the basic story arc of nearly every medical TV show.

In *The Citadel*[1] by AJ Cronin (1937), Andrew Manson, a young doctor newly arrived at a hillside community in Wales, challenges a colleague when asked to countersign an order to section a 'mad' patient. Emry Hughes has 'been acting strangely lately, getting into trouble at the mine, losing his memory. He had turned quarrelsome and violent. He had set upon his wife with a carving knife.' Andrew looks at the man, notes his swollen legs, his coarse facial appearance, and refuses. He starts Mr Hughes on thyroid hormone, watches him closely, and within a week the patient is back to his old self. His family takes him back, forever grateful. The psychosis was physical, due to a deficiency, and wholly curable. Andrew was right! Every junior doctor who has started work in a new hospital and made a good impression on a ward round will have experienced the same, brief feeling of elation.

These 'wins' occur more often than mistakes, but they do not leave the same legacy in the mind of the doctor. It could be argued that wins should not be regarded as wins at all, but as normal service. Are we not trained and paid to be correct all the time? Perhaps for this reason, doctors are not good at celebrating success. Many hospitals in the UK record errors by encouraging staff to fill out a 'DATIX' (an electronic repository of patient safety incidents). Now we also have the GREATIX, so that we can notify the hospital when a member of staff does something particularly well. The idea has not really taken off; our minds, and emotions, are more easily drawn to error. And to blame.

Dame Jane Elizabeth Dacre, DBE (president of the Royal College of Physicians from 2014 to 2018) promoted the Twitter hashtag **#medicineisgreat**. Having read this book, you may disagree. With the 'great' comes pain and suffering. Somehow, young doctors must use stores of positive experiences to support them in times of stress. The sources of positive energy are different for everyone. For me, that energy comes from making correct diagnoses and in hastening recovery through practical procedures. So why not start this book with a success?

DOI: 10.1201/9781003189824-1

One of my proudest moments occurred just 18 months after qualifying as a doctor. A young man called Andrew came to the hospital with numb legs. He was otherwise completely well. There seemed to be a level halfway up his back above which sensation was normal, but below that he could not feel a pinprick. Examining each side of the body, I realised that it was more subtle than that. On the left, Andrew could not feel sharp pain, whereas on the right he could. But on the right, he could not pick up the vibrations of a tuning fork when its base was pressed against a prominent bone. It was not so long ago that I had studied neurology, and I was still in the books most nights while I prepared for an important exam. In my mind I saw a figure, a drawing of a man with a line down the middle, demarcating two zones of sensory change. Could this really be Brown-Sequard syndrome, a diagnostic 'zebra'?[2]

In this condition, a spinal cord tumour presses on the long nerves, causing loss of sensation to pain, temperature and light touch on one side of the body, and reduced perception of vibration, positional sense and deep touch on the other. It requires patience and skill to detect those signs. I struck the tuning fork against my knee yet again, checked and rechecked, then borrowed another doctor's medical handbook (there was no easy access to the internet in the late 1990s). Confident in my findings, I sat down to write my impression on the clerking paper. If I was wrong, I would look over-confident, too wrapped up in small print rarities and eponymous conditions. Only an MRI scan would tell, and that could not be done until a specialist had seen the patient. Next day I went to the ward and took out Andrew's file. When I saw *'Agree Brown-Sequard'* underneath my own entry, written floridly in brown fountain pen ink by a consultant neurologist, my chest filled. I had been a doctor for less than two years. It couldn't get better than this.

I was right.

1.2 Slick

Practical procedures are the currency of progression as a junior doctor. The more you conquer and become independent at doing them, the higher your sense of self-esteem. At first it is the simple blood test, then the venous cannula ('venflon') and the arterial blood gas sample. These teach you what human skin and tissue feel like when punctured, and develop the art of visualising where a needle is headed once it has sunk beneath the surface of the body. But the big-ticket procedures were lumbar punctures (LP) and central line insertions.

LPs look horrible. You ask the patient to curl up on their side in the bed, identify a gap between two vertebrae, sterilise the skin, anaesthetise the tissue, then pass a very long, very thin needle through skin, fat, tendon, dura… until there is a little give and precious, clear fluid runs out through the needle. Then you hold a sterile pot in fingers that are trembling with tension beneath the needle's hub to collect the drops.

I was getting on well with the procedure. My finger could find the right spot straight away, without the elaborate tracing of landmarks and imaginary lines across the back that I had been taught to do at first. I was slick. A friend of mine was faring less well; one afternoon I overheard her consultant say,

'Look, Nicky, this is a neuro job. There are three or four LPs to do every Thursday afternoon. You *can't* be missing them like this.' What a way to teach!

I was working in casualty. An elderly patient with fever, headache and neck stiffness arrived. He needed an LP. My registrar asked if I was happy to do it, and I nodded. I had seven or eight under my belt. She left me alone.

I prepared Mr Sharif. His back was stiff from arthritis, and I could not feel a nice wide gap between the two vertebrae. But the site was easy to locate, and I swiftly confirmed it using the line between promontories made by the pelvic bones. Then I infiltrated the anaesthetic and started to press the needle through the tissue. More than half on the needle was inside the patient when I felt the scrape of metal on the bone. He moved. I withdrew, changed my angle and tried again. Bone, again. No fluid.

The curtain moved behind me, and I sensed someone looking down at me.

'What are you doing?' It was my registrar.

'What do you mean?' I replied, without turning round.

'Stop!' she said, anxiety in her voice. I was bewildered. She leaned down to the level of my ear and whispered,

'You're *miles* out.' Then she pulled on gloves and located the true landmarks. The bony lumps I had used as landmarks without much more than a glance were his arthritic hip bones. She was right, I was two inches too low. My needle was exploring an area well below the spinal canal, where the nerves spread out to the lower body. No wonder all I couldn't find any fluid. I dreaded to think what it had pierced.

My confidence was wrecked. The registrar knew me; she knew I was generally competent. She took me outside the cubicle and, in a tone that was both kind and uncompromising, said,

'You've got to be sure. You've got to be a hundred percent sure.'

I followed Mr Sharrif's progress, nervous that he would be paralysed due to a severed nerve at the base of his spine. But he got out of bed and walked; I was reprieved. More importantly, I never took a short cut with a lumbar puncture, or any other practical procedure, again. They teach those imaginary lines and landmarks for a reason.

1.3 Shock

With growing experience comes independence, and with independence comes the need to make decisions about when to ask for help. One night, I admitted a patient with low blood pressure. He had a fever, and there was evidence that he had a kidney infection. I kept him in the resuscitation bay ('resus') and gave fluids through the cannula. In those days, there was no pressure to move patients out of casualty within four hours[3], and the registrar was off on the wards or sleeping. It was me in charge, 18 months out of medical school. Help was available if I called for it, but nobody was going to pop in just in case.

With a litre of fluid, Mr Collins' blood pressure rose a few notches, but 15 minutes later, it was down again to a worrying level. I gave another litre. Same effect. I saw some other patients and came back to him. A third litre went in. Not only was the blood pressure low, but he wasn't producing any urine either. This meant his kidneys were shutting down. His fever had reduced but his blood tests appeared to be in keeping with an infection. I began to think about referring to the ICU, where he could receive an infusion of noradrenaline, a drug that tightens the blood vessels and raises the blood pressure. I knew where I was going with this man. One or two more litres, then I would make the call. No point calling ICU too soon; the registrar would just tell me to give another fluid challenge.

It was 5 AM. The fifth litre was nearly complete. Five litres are a lot of extra fluid. We carry five litres of blood in our arteries and veins, so I had doubled this volume with crystalloid (a water-based fluid). As I approached him, I noticed that he was wearing an oxygen mask attached to a high-flow re-breather bag.

'What happened?' I asked the nurse in charge of resus.

'He suddenly got short of breath.'

I listened to his lungs with my stethoscope. There were florid crackles, suggestive of pulmonary oedema. Fluid was leaking out of his lung capillaries into the air sacs. He was coughing, and there was white froth on his lips.

I stopped the fluid and drew arterial blood to measure the oxygen level accurately. 10 minutes later I was back, with the slip of paper that the blood gas machine had produced. His oxygen was critically low. I prescribed a diuretic, to make him pass urine quickly. But it was going to take too long. I called intensive care. 10 minutes later, the ICU doctor arrived in the company of my registrar (not the same one who had observed my rotten lumbar puncture). She was clearly annoyed that the first she had heard of a crisis in casualty was from the ICU doctor. He quickly assessed Mr Collins and made arrangements to intubate the patient there and then. The only way to get oxygen into him was to put him on a ventilator. Sarah, the registrar, was standing nearby holding Mr Collins' heart tracing, or ECG. She looked over at me, her brow knitted.

'Phil. Why did you give five litres of fluid to a guy in heart failure?'

'What. It's septic shock. Refractory to fluids... isn't it?'

'I doubt it. Look at this.' She pointed out subtle features in the ECG showing that Mr Collins' heart was damaged. The changes were subtle, for me. For her, they were glaring. The back of his heart, hidden from the electrodes on his chest, had infarcted. Then she looked at the chest x-ray performed shortly after he had been admitted. There were tiny lines near the edges of the lungs, consistent with an early build-up of fluid. I had nearly drowned an already drowning man.

'He needed dobutamine on CCU.'

Of course, he did. Dobutamine increases the contractile power of the ventricles. I knew this. I could handle cardiac failure. But you must make the diagnosis before you can treat it.

'Damn. I'm sorry.'

'It's okay,' she said, as uncomfortable as I. 'But when a patient doesn't respond, you've got to ask yourself why.'

I nodded, embarrassed. I was tempted to point to the 10 other patients I had successfully diagnosed and treated overnight without any advice or assistance. But that would have been to miss the point. She was right. I had held on too long, dead set on proving my diagnosis, and to the detriment of the patient.

1.4 Pride

Years later, working on an ICU, I admitted a young female patient with liver failure called Maghadi Padam. The liver produces many essential substances, including glucose, enzymes and clotting factors. Without the latter, the blood thins and if there is any bleeding, internally or externally, it does not tend to stop.

I was the only doctor on the unit. Each patient was attended by a nurse. Nearly all were asleep, in medically induced comas. In this way, their bodily functions could be controlled by machines, and by us; their breathing, their blood pressure, their kidneys and their brains. I was seeing another patient at the far end of the unit when a voice called out,

'Doctor! Doctor! Bed 3!' The new patient. Only 34 years old. Her liver had collapsed shortly after giving birth due to eclampsia. I knew that she was heading towards a liver transplant, if she managed to survive the next 24 hours.

I ran to bed 3. The alarms rang, and her oxygen saturation reading flashed – 72%. 90% was the bare minimum. Her ventilator alarms were also ringing. The machine was struggling to push oxygen down the endotracheal tube and into the lungs. The resistance was too high. I took the stethoscope that hung from an infusion stand by the bed and pressed the diaphragm to her chest wall, first the left, then the right. There was no air entering the right lung. Then I percussed the right lung; it was stony dull. This meant the usual air-filled space under the ribs was full of fluid. That fluid could only be one thing – blood.

Her oxygen saturation had fallen to 68%. Her heart would not keep going for long at this level. I had seen it before. After three or four minutes, the tracing would slow, the blood pressure would collapse and cardiac arrest would ensue.

I attached a needle to a 10 ml syringe, slid it between two ribs and pulled the plunger. Dark blood filled the cylinder. Diagnosis confirmed. Saturations 64%.

'Chest drain.'

The nurse knew exactly what I meant. She fetched a steel trolley and began to collect the necessary equipment. I ran to the storeroom at the far end of the unit and grabbed the drain, the tubing and the bottle into which the blood would drain. I glanced at my watch. It was 6:30 AM. The windows were brightening.

Back beside Maghadi (who knew nothing and felt nothing), I smeared pink chlorhexidine onto the skin, injected some anaesthetic (by force of habit, wondering if this was necessary) and made a one-inch-long incision. This was generous, but I did not want to be struggling. I pressed a gloved finger into the wound, then made the hole deeper by opening the blunt forceps between the ribs, tearing at the tissue and the muscle. I could soon feel the out pleura, one of the membranes that surrounds the lung. The blood was collecting between the outer and inner layer. I rubbed the outer pleura with the tip of my index finger, trying to tear a hole in it. It would not give way. I took out the finger and pushed the forceps in deep. The metal nose of the forceps succeeded in pushing the fibres apart, because when I replaced my finger I could feel a defect. I worked on this until it gave way. Warm blood surrounded my finger, then flowed along the tunnel that I had created and out of the patient. It was under pressure, and two streams of blood poured away on each side of my finger, covering her skin, running over the sheet, spilling off the bed and onto the floor. I took the chest drain, supported by a metal trocar, and slid it through the gap, guided by my finger. Blood immediately filled the attached tubing and began to fill the two litre bottle that stood on the floor. After two minutes, I had to clamp the tube and empty the bottle. Her saturations had risen to 75%. It was working. With a needle and silk thread, I secured the drain to her skin and covered the area with a strong dressing. On no account could that drain fall out.

Saturation 82%. Blood pressure improved as well. My God, it was working.

The bottle was emptied for a second time, and now the flow was easing. I listened again with the stethoscope: air was rushing in and out of the right lung in time with the ventilator. Everything was getting better.

Now I removed the surgical gown and gloves, washed up a little and sat down to document everything in cool medical terms. I heard footsteps approaching and looked round. It was my consultant, arriving early before the handover ward round. She poked her head into the cubicle, and grimaced. The floor hadn't been mopped yet.

'Everything alright in here, Phil?'

'Oh yes. Just a little ventilation issue, sorted for now, I think. I'll tell you at handover.'

This was glory. Quiet glory. There is a clip from the great American medical drama *ER* that was shared as a GIF on social media, used to signify self-congratulation. The arrogant, brilliant surgeon Benton walks along a corridor and springs into a victorious pose, shooting one hand forward, punching the air. He knows he has achieved something remarkable, and that he is at the top of his game. That's how I felt after saving Maghadi's life with the chest drain.

Six weeks later, I was covering the ICU again. A young male patient called Abraham had been admitted during the day. I was not very pleased to be told that he needed 'to be lined up', i.e., to have tubes inserted in the veins and arteries for monitoring, haemofiltration (a kind of kidney dialysis) and drug infusions. Three lines. Not normally a problem. The complicating factor here was that leukaemia had wiped out his bone marrow, and he was not producing any platelets. These are as important, perhaps more so, as clotting factors in stopping bleeding. Nevertheless, he was receiving two 'pools' (bags), and the platelet level should be above the safety margin when I came to do the lines.

I started with two lines in the groin, and they went well. The third I decided to insert in the neck. This was a large line, thick enough to allow a good flow of blood into and out of the haemofilter. He was asleep, on the ventilator, completely unaware.

I sterilised the neck. I identified the site of the internal jugular vein. I injected local anaesthetic. Then I took the seeker needle and passed it through the skin, down into the region of the vein. Blood flashed up into the cylinder.

'Shit!' I muttered. The blood was bright red and came out with enough force to push the syringe's plunger out without any help from me. I had hit the carotid. This was rare for me [nowadays we are trained in the use of ultrasound to make sure we do not miss]. But never mind, I knew what to do. Press hard for five minutes. This delay would impact on the rest of my tasks, but it was early still, barely 9 PM. I had the whole night to go around the other patients.

After five minutes I took my finger off the puncture site, but blood welled up. I was not surprised. His coagulation was off, we knew that. The platelets we had transfused might not function as well as his own would have. I pressed for ten minutes this time.

Finger off. Blood. Coming up from the major neck artery as swiftly as before. There had been no change. He was incapable of clotting. A familiar feeling came over me. Like wandering into the sea and feeling the slope accelerate beneath your feet. The water laps at your chest, then hits your chin, and a current is pulling at you. You look back at the shore, but nobody is looking in your direction.

'Could you hold this for a while?' I asked the nurse. She stood next to me and pressed two fingers to the wad of gauze. Despite the pressure I had been maintaining, the gauze was soaked. The blood was getting watery. I asked for a second nurse to check the patient's haemoglobin level on the nearby blood gas machine, while I went to make a phone call. My consultant advised me to contact the haematologist on call. I did so. They offered every clotting product in the lab. Arrangements were made to deliver them to the unit. While I held the phone to one ear, the second nurse put the blood gas report down on the desk. I scanned it quickly. *'Haemoglobin – 5 g/dL'.* Abraham had lost much more blood than I had seen coming out through the skin.

'Doctor!' called the first nurse. I rushed to the cubicle. 'Look' she said, pointing along Abraham's body. There was a huge bruise tracking from the neck, along the collarbone and down the chest wall. Blood was seeping out of the artery and under the skin, pints of it.

Now the alarms began to sound. Blood pressure – low; heart rate – high.

'What's happening, Phil?' asked the nurse in charge. She roamed the unit fighting fires and solving problems, like me. She had seen most things. Not this.

'He's bleeding out... through one needle puncture. I hadn't even used the introducer needle. It was just a green needle.' Already, the feeling of panic was manifesting itself in excuses. But I genuinely did not understand how a green needle could lead to this.

'Keep the pressure on; ask someone else to do it if you're getting tired, sorry. I have to make another call.'

I rang the consultant. He was despondent. I got the feeling he had seen this before, and that he knew what the outcome was going to be.

'What about vascular surgery – could they operate? Or interventional radiology?' He was not enthusiastic, but yes, I could try. The new clotting products had arrived and were running in. I hoped that they would help the blood to coagulate. We gave blood to support the haemoglobin. I would not stop. He was in his twenties. My phone calls to the other specialties resulted in sympathetic refusals to intervene. I understood. There was no operation for this.

I entered the cubicle. The bruise was even larger, more red than blue, fresh. I could feel the bogginess under the skin.

'I've turned up the norad,' explained the nurse in charge. She was camped here now. 'Do you think we should set limits?'

I was shocked. Setting limits was to admit that we were losing this struggle.

'And the family,' she added. 'We need to call the family.'

So here we were. A patient who had been admitted with hope was now going to die on my watch, because the needle I had passed hit the artery instead of the vein. I nodded.

'Yes. You're right.' And to the nurse who was assigned to the patient. 'Please keep the pressure on.' She looked unimpressed. It hadn't worked, it wasn't working now, it wasn't going to work.

Abraham's mother was accepting. I realised that she had been prepared for the worst as he was being transferred to intensive care. Numerous organs were failing already. But I had to explain that this bleeding started with the needle. She did not shout or blame me. It was part of the overall situation.

We kept him alive until sunrise, using many litres of blood and clotting factors, but in the end his heart stopped.

I left the hospital after handover in quiet shock. I gazed out of the train window and looked at my clean, pale hands. They could do just as much damage as good. If I was to choose a medical specialty that involved invasive procedures, I was going to have to get used to this dreadful feeling.

1.5 Listen

i. Doctors make many decisions each day, and some of them are bound to be wrong. The important cognitive steps are diagnosis, prognosis and management plan. If the first is wrong, the second and third will also be wrong. If the first two are right, it is still possible to mess up the third.

Mr Braithwaite had a swallowing problem. He had already undergone an internal examination, and nothing serious was found. The first doctor thought there was something wrong with the way the muscles in his gullet were working.

Some months later, in my clinic this time, he asked to have another examination, an endoscopy. I declined, knowing that it would do no good. His symptoms were the same; there was no earthly point in visualising the area again. He came to see me again, two months later, and asked the same question.

'Why not?', he asked. I explained, we don't just go and check things for the sake of it. The diagnosis was clear. I had a plan for him. I referred him to a specialist in that area. I knew he wasn't happy with me, and I thought hard about my refusal. But I decided to stand by the principle. It just isn't right to arrange an investigation just because a patient wants one.

Two months later I ran a finger down the list of new cancer patients to be discussed in our multi-disciplinary meeting. I saw his name – Alan Braithwaite. And a brief summary:

OGD: ulcerated friable lesion at 30 cm

Histology: moderately differentiated squamous cell carcinoma

CT: bulky concentric thickening from level carina-GOJ: extramural invasion, 90% contact aorta: para tracheal LN suspicious, left gastric & small

Provisional stage: T4N3M0

Let's break down this hyper-technical summary:

OGD – oesophagogastroduodenoscopy, the term for endoscopy, or a camera test. Somebody had arranged one for him without me knowing. *Ulcerated friable lesion* – that could mean only one thing; cancer. *Histology* – they had taken a biopsy, and it had proven cancer. *CT* – a computed tomography scan; *bulky*; *contacting the aorta* – i.e., a tumour touching the great central blood vessel that runs down the middle of the body. *Provisional* stage – T4; the highest. *N3*; lymph nodes involved.

Cancer, advanced and well beyond surgery. Terminal disease.

Oh, no.

My throat tightened. With a little digging, the full story was revealed. Unknown to me, Mr Braithwaite had been admitted to a ward with new symptoms. Food was getting completely stuck, and he had lost 7 kg in weight. A tumour was found, already advanced, growing just above the stomach. It had been too small to find at the time of the first endoscopy, but it had been growing larger during those two appointments. Two wasted appointments. He would have done better to see somebody else, somebody who listened to him. If I had acquiesced to his request, it would have been found earlier.

My memory of that man was laced with regret, self-criticism, and a little fear (Why did I not listen to him? Will I be accused?). But looking back, every decision was defensible. You don't investigate unless there are new symptoms, different features... you just don't. Although I failed, I didn't do anything demonstrably wrong. So somehow, through a labour of sophistry, I was able to conclude that I was both right and wrong. My decisions were defensible, but my diagnosis was wrong. For the patient, who had no interest in the complexities of my mind, the subtleties of diagnosis or even the obligation we have to use medical resources responsibly, I was 100% wrong.

What lesson could I draw? It was a simple one. Listen, and when a patient asks the same question more than once, reconsider. They know their body better than you do. They are persisting for a reason.

ii. Two weeks into my first job as a consultant, I learned that this lesson does not just apply to patients. Colleagues have questions too, and the thoughts that underpin those sometimes oblique queries need to be drawn out.

I was conducting a ward round. A new patient with alcoholic cirrhosis had been transferred to the ward. My senior house officer (SHO) presented the case.

'He's been triggering all night, low blood pressure. Down to 80 systolic.'

'He's septic, you said.'

'Yes, spontaneous bacterial peritonitis[4], confirmed.'

'He's passing urine; he looks alert. Lactate's normal. Give him more time, he should skate through without needing vasopressors.'

Later that day, my SHO found me in endoscopy.

'He's not picking up. We'll need to adjust the alarm parameters if we don't want to be bleeped about his BP every thirty minutes.'

'This is what cirrhotics do, run low BPs, dilated circulations, even without sepsis. A bit more filling, another couple of days of antibiotics and he should turn around.'

Next morning she came to my office; the registrar was away.

'I'm worried. Sodium's down, BP is still poor. And he's got a rash, all over his trunk. It's blue.'

'But he's talking, reading the paper, walking to the toilet. I passed him on the ward this morning. I'm not too concerned about him.'

'But he's just not right...'

A brief stab of annoyance interrupted my continued reassurances – yes, we're all worried about him, but get on with it!

On the third morning I was called to the ICU. My patient lay dying, his skin mottled, a cardiac output monitor confirming that his heart was not pumping properly. An echocardiogram had been performed that morning, and it demonstrated that its muscles were weak and barely moving. He had been displaying signs of severe alcoholic cardiomyopathy from day one, and I had missed it. My SHO had never seen a case before, but she had sensed it, the wrongness... I didn't hear her, because I was sure I knew more. When she insisted, I became irritated. I did not listen.

1.6 Patterns

There is another important voice in this triad of doctor, patient and colleague. Your own. When a patient does not respond as well as you expected them to, that voice begins to nag. That voice was suppressed when I overloaded with fluid the patient who had suffered a heart attack. In the case that follows, there were ample opportunities to hear that voice, yet still I did not. I was too busy cutting my patient to fit the Procrustean couch.

1.6.1 Day 1

There are not many occasions when you recognise the clues, feel bold enough to make a diagnosis and see admiration in the eyes of your colleagues – some of whom didn't even know who you were.

The patient came in with fever and was referred to me as just another pneumonia or a urinary infection, but I noticed that one of his blood results was unusually high. The eosinophils. This led me to ask about his travel history, because these cells often go up when there are parasites in the system. And indeed, he had travelled, a fact that no one else had thought to ask. I looked up the country in which he had spent time and worked out what sort of parasites could be involved. But I knew which one already. The symptoms seemed to fit what he was describing, to the letter. Fever, abdominal pain, some weight loss and especially breathing difficulties that he had developed just before coming to hospital. It all fit.

So, I looked up the treatment, called the pharmacist to make sure we had it in stock and prescribed it. By the end of the day, he was already feeling better. It made all the study seem worthwhile. But it was a special memory that served me so well today. I had seen a patient just like this one during my elective (a period spent abroad during medical training). I even wrote about it in the report that we had to hand in, so it stuck in my brain. Strongyloides. I suppose, over a whole career, many such images and stories will find a place in my memory, to be retrieved at a later date. Nothing wasted, they all find a niche. A *good* day.

1.6.2 Day 2

I went straight in to see him as soon as I arrived at the hospital. He was grateful and asked how long it would take him to get better. I said I would refer him to the tropical disease specialist, as they see more of this sort of thing. And of course, I explained that we needed to confirm the diagnosis, even though I was pretty sure about it. I reviewed his blood tests and saw that his kidneys weren't working so well. He must have got very dehydrated before he came in. His breathing had settled slightly, but he was still struggling. I didn't want to come across as an expert, because I have only ever seen one other person with this. But he's on the right track.

1.6.3 Day 3

I was disappointed. His kidneys were worse, despite the fluids that I prescribed. My consultant didn't have any new ideas; she was happy to go along with my explanation. But she was keen to see confirmation of the diagnosis. The antibody tests will take days, as they must be done in London. She asked me whether it could be any other parasite, or any other type of infection, full stop. Perhaps she doesn't quite trust my impression. It made me think and reflect. But I've seen the list of parasites, and none of the others that he might have acquired in Africa presents like this. So I suggested that we push on with the current treatment. It worked last time, I explained.

1.6.4 Day 4

Weird. He appeared confused. This parasite can affect the brain, though. I spent 45 minutes on the phone trying to get through to a tropical disease expert, to see what they thought. They agreed, yes, strongyloides can go into the brain. I arranged a scan, and it's happening after hours tonight. The anti-parasitic agent we're giving him will kick in soon, I thought.

1.6.5 Day 5

I went to see him, but he wasn't there. I ran into another SHO in the corridor who had been on call overnight and he told me he'd been transferred to the ICU. I almost ran. When I got there, I found him unconscious, on a ventilator. He was surrounded by other doctors. There was a neurologist, examining his eyes. I asked what was going on. He had blown a pupil, I was told. It didn't make sense. I saw a nurse returning from one of the computers. She was shaking her head. 'What!' shouted one of the other consultants, a rheumatologist. 'They must have done it!' he said. I faded into the background, but I continued to listen. What angered him was the fact that during the patient's entire admission, no one had sent off a vasculitis screen. As soon as I heard that word, vasculitis, my heart dropped and the muscles in my legs grew weak. I had to sit down behind the nurses' station. I realised that I had made a huge mistake. For vasculitis is another main reason for eosinophils to be raised. I knew immediately what the diagnosis was – Churg–Strauss syndrome. I had missed it completely.

1.6.6 Day 9

I met with my clinical supervisor. I had asked for the meeting. I told her what happened. I could tell that she thought my mistake was a bit stupid. She asked me what my thought processes were on the day the patient came in. I explained the whole story, how it rung bells in my mind, how the words that he used, and the clinical examination findings, had taken me back to a vivid moment in my training. And I had questioned the data, and I had tested the hypothesis, and it all seemed to fit.
    'But what about the differential diagnosis?' she asked.
    'I... I...'
    'Did you develop one?'
    'I did, I think. I'm n...'
    'Did you write it down, in the clerking? Did you test for anything else?'
    'I didn't think I needed to. It was so clear.'
    'Well, to be fair, the patient saw a lot of other people, and more senior than you, before he got really ill. No one really challenged the diagnosis. There's a lesson for all of us. But it shows you the power of a positive diagnosis. Especially one that appears to be supported with confidence. You're a junior doctor, but you see how much weight people give the opinion of anybody who seems sure of themselves. Yes, diagnoses should be challenged by more senior doctors as they review patients, but it is not uncommon for them to defer to the opinion of the first doctor who really got

their teeth into the case. And that was you. You made a plan, it made sense, the patient even got a little bit better at first. Sometimes, I think, there is really one chance to set things into motion in the right direction, and that's on the first day of admission. It's a big responsibility. Am I making you feel any better?' She smiled. Then she asked, 'What would you do differently next time?'

'I won't be so confident.'

'That would be a shame, if you are right.'

'Well, if I really think I'm right, I will make my case confidently. But I will make sure there are caveats, and that other avenues aren't closed off right at the beginning. Perhaps in this case, because he had raised eosinophils, he should've seen a rheumatologist anyway, even if I really thought he had an infection.'

'I'll tell you what I take away from this. The power of anecdote. In your mind there was a clear story, and narrative that you had seen played out before, one with a happy ending. You were sucked back into that memory. If you're like me, your memory works best when it's embedded in stories. But I guess that might be at a disadvantage, if you can't stand back and approach each case with pure objectivity. Attack each case with fresh eyes, but use the stories that you recollect to remind you of all the possibilities.'

'I hear you.'

'And one more thing. The Procrustean Bed.'

'The what?'

'His confusion. It challenged your hypothesis, it didn't make sense, but you rationalised it, and made it fit your idea – a parasite in the brain. Procrustes chopped or stretched travellers who encountered him until they fit the size of his bed. You not only fell into the trap of anecdotal memory, but you tailored your interpretation of the data so as to support it…'

'There is one more thing.'

'Tell me.'

'I was pleased with myself, on the first day. I felt elated to make a difficult diagnosis.'

'That may be the most valuable lesson of all. It's seductive, the warmth that being right gives you. But don't worry, you'll experience enough reverses in your career to learn that pride is never to be entertained. I think you've learnt enough from this particular case, don't you! How is he, by the way?'

'Better, thanks.'

It was a good meeting.

That meeting never happened.

Those words are the product of a meeting that took place in my own head.

Lesson: rare cases don't necessarily teach good medicine. I may never see a case of Churg– Strauss again. The good to come out of this was in the reflection, about making positive diagnoses, about cutting and stretching the story to fit a mental model. If there had been a supervisor to talk to back then (the absence of senior doctors was the reason I was left in charge for so long), we might have had that conversation. Now, as a consultant, I make very sure that I am available to have those conversations when my juniors make mistakes. Something good may have come out of it.

1.7 Ignorant

Diagnosis and management are easy, compared to making a prognosis. This requires us to look into the future, and the human body is too complex a machine to allow complete confidence in our predictions.

A very sick patient with liver failure came in. He struggled, we struggled; he responded to intensive care support, we felt satisfied that our decision to advocate for aggressive treatment was the right one. He deteriorated; we isolated the infection. We talked the family through it and suggested that we not give up yet. He fluctuated, weakening a little with each reverse, until... weeks later, he died. All that hope. All that work. The 'numbers', at one stage, had looked better. But that is the nature of the disease. Unexpected complications. Hidden infections. Sudden ruptures.

The shapes and lines of that patient's clinical course remained etched in my mind when, months later, I recognised an almost identical scenario. Her liver function looked the same during the first week. Her slide into an ICU bed occurred over a similar interval. I was 'guarded' in my prognosis, but I knew what was going to happen here. I knew. The road home presented too many traps and potholes for her body to negotiate, given the advanced nature of her disease. Any and each of them could kill her in a few hours. As time passed, her clinical course described the usual sinusoidal curve. The downslopes were not catastrophic enough to justify withdrawal, and the upward gradients were not sufficiently sustained to launch a bid for convalescence.

We reacted to each complication with urgency. Our policy was unchanged – treat, support, save. But my heart was not really in it. I did not have hope. I know I communicated that to trainees. Those muttered opinions as we walked out of intensive care. But at no point did we hesitate or withhold. And time passed.

Until... she returned to the ward. She turned the corner. She had climbed far enough up the hill for the swirling, sucking mists of death to no longer have a hold on her. Then she went home.

A trainee asked, 'You know _____? I thought you said the chances of her surviving were...' I stopped her there and turned the case into an occasion to teach about uncertainty.

Is it a 'survival gene'? Poor science. Then what? We do not know. Probably, luck is involved. When such large unknowns are involved, when the rules that underlie our attempted predictions appear unfixed, pattern recognition can lead to erroneous conclusions. Sometimes it's better just to treat, support, stand back, and try not to outthink the disease... hoping that they turn the corner.

To avoid making mistakes it is necessary to admit ignorance. My first midnight ward round in the ICU, still inexperienced. The patient in cubicle 4 was deteriorating. His oxygen requirement was maximal; the pressure settings on the ventilator had crept up. His lungs were stiffening, be it due to infection, fluid overload or a tense abdomen... I could not be sure. The last blood gas was dismal.

The nurse in charge, Tom, looked at me expectantly. I looked hard at the ventilator settings, at the squared off curve on the display that signified the depth and duration of each artificial breath. I had no idea. Tom was still looking at me.

'What do you want to do?' he asked.

I scoured my shallow memory for solutions: 'Call the consultant, I guess.'

He raised an eyebrow. Wrong answer, clearly. Then I pulled the joker, the card I had used so many times before – as a junior house officer on the wards confronted by a severely agitated patient, as a short-lived infectious disease trainee in the micro lab, on the coronary care unit when presented with an horrific arrhythmia –

'So, err... what do you normally do in this situation?'

Translation: Help me out here.

Tom whispered, 'Do you want to consider a recruitment manoeuvre?'

Yes! The tunnel of my ignorance was illuminated. I considered it with quiet dignity, as though weighing up the pros and cons of this well known, if exotic, option.

'Err, yes... good idea. They use that... here... do they?'

'All the time.'

I nodded. I had a plan.

'Right. Let's do it.' Firm. Confident.

Tom's arms were folded. There was no humour in his eyes. This was a serious situation. My hand moved towards the ventilator, slowly, automatically, under obligation rather than conscious control. Its fingers did not know what to do once they reached the control panel. The hand slowed, stretching the moment in time. Was that a smile tugging at the corner of Tom's usually inscrutable mouth? The reprieve ended.

'And err... what do you usually start with...?'

'Have you done a recruitment manoeuvre before?' asked Tom.

'You inflate the lungs, put up the...the...'

'The PEEP.'

'Yes, the PEEP. For...'

'A minute.'

'Yeah, right. And PEEP of...'

'Whatever you like.'

'25, 30?'

'40.'

'Yeah, good. Then you...'

'That's it.'

'Yes, of course. Good. Right, let's... do you want to do it?'

Tom shook his head. He did not say it, but the movement was a silent version of 'You're the doctor... you do it.'

My finger hovered over the relevant dial. Tom watched. This was his idea. He had seen it done a hundred, perhaps a thousand times. He should be doing this. But this was an intervention. I had to take responsibility for it, I had to deliver it. I dialled up the pressure and pressed the button that kept it raised despite the alarms, forcing the ventilator to inflate those lungs and open up the air sacs that had become clogged up and useless.

Nothing bad happened. In fact, it worked.

Next morning, I handed over each patient to the newly arrived consultant and the day team. We entered cubicle 4. I explained how the patient had deteriorated.

'And what did you do?' asked the consultant. She was scrutinising the settings, making a quick assessment as to the seriousness of the situation. Tom was not there; he was sorting something else out along the unit.

'Recruitment manoeuvre.'

She looked at me blankly for a moment. God damn it, Tom! It was your idea. I knew it, I knew it was dangerous... I remembered now, it had been associated with pneumothoraces, burst lungs... I should have called. The consultant glanced at the last set of blood gases and nodded.

'Good. Good knowledge.'

We moved onto cubicle 5. My mouth opened to say, 'Actually it was Tom's idea...' but the moment had passed.

Tired and anxious to get home to sleep before the next night shift, I passed Tom on the way out.

'Thanks for the advice, Tom.'

He looked surprised. It was nothing. This was a large part of his professional life. Sharing the knowledge of countless shifts with new, green doctors who by virtue of their medical qualifications were permitted to do things to patients, even though they barely understood them. He shared that knowledge freely, to the benefit of patients, yes, but also to the benefit of those doctors who were destined to move on after a few months, their experience augmented, magpie-like.

1.8 Stop

The patient's heart had stopped. She was dead. We were trying to resuscitate her. I was leading the crash team.

'Let's do another cycle, and then I think we'll stop. There's been no electrical activity since we started...all agree?'

The situation looked hopeless. She had been suffering from pneumonia and was elderly. In retrospect, she should probably have had a DNACPR order.[5] But it was too late for that now. We were doing chest compressions, trying the cannulate veins in which the too dark blood seemed to be thickening already.

A cardiology registrar entered the cubicle pushing a portable echocardiography machine.

'I'm just going to take a look, see if there's any ventricular activity.'

I interjected: 'We're just about to call it. She's dead, unfortunately. We've been going for 20 minutes in asystole.'[6]

'But you haven't excluded all reversible causes yet. What about tamponade? She's anti-coagulated.'

'There's no reason to suspect tamponade, no instrumentation, no electrical activity on the monitor...'

'It will only take a couple of minutes. My consultant will want to know before you stop resuscitation.'

'What! No! I'm running this arrest, we've given four shots of adrenaline, and the line is flat. She is dead. I'm not going to have this woman subjected to another 10 minutes of CPR while you do an echo and go and call your consultant.'

'It's protocol on the cardiology ward.'

'She's only on this ward because the others were full. She's under general medicine.'

'That's two minutes,' called one of the nurses. He had been counting off the seconds between electric shocks. The time had come for another electric shock, or... for us to call it a day. I spoke,

'Okay, what's the rhythm...asystole, not compatible with a pulse. Let's stop. Stop compressions.'

'I'm calling my consultant,' said the cardiologist.

Sternly, controlling my irritation, I said, 'Do so. At no point in the life support algorithm does it mention echocardiograms and phone calls to consultants. We're stopping.'

I walked away, emboldened. Yes, I wasn't immune to making mistakes myself, but I would stand my ground when I saw that one was just about to happen.

1.9 Wait

The dullest medical job I ever did was admitting patients who were due to attend for a TURP[7]. In this procedure, the inner lining of the prostate gland is scraped away to improve the flow of urine from the bladder. It is done with an inflexible metal camera inserted into the penis, under anaesthetic. I saw a few, and I didn't like it. However, like many men, it will probably be my turn someday.

A stream of relatively healthy men sat in the waiting room, while one by one I listened to their hearts and lungs and arranged blood tests. If all was well, I signed them off as fit for the surgery. Usually, I could tell if someone was fit as soon as they sat in the chair. It was a most mundane job.

I came into work one morning to a frosty reception. One of the TURP patients had been transferred to intensive care. He collapsed after the operation with low oxygen levels and ended up on a ventilator. His chest x-ray showed a complete 'white out'. His right lung was full of fluid.

The consultant had the medical notes. He was looking at my diagram of the lungs, and the big tick that I had made through them, indicating 'lungs clear'. He knew me, a little. He trusted me. I was reliable.

'Did you listen to his lungs?' he asked.

'Yes. Definitely.' Did I? I know I had. Often tempted to skip the examination, I could never cross the line of writing something in the notes that was untrue. We had been told many times that medical notes are a 'legal document'.

'Well, it's very odd,' he said. With these mild words he was saying, 'I don't believe you, but I'm not going to crucify you.'

I dragged myself through another dull day on the urology ward. I felt rubbish. But I could not explain it. Had I failed to listen to his lungs properly? Or perhaps a devilish aspect of my personality had indeed skipped the examination. Christ!

Two days later, the same consultant attended a handover round. Insouciantly, he said,

'Oh, by the way, that fluid. It was glycine. We flush in gallons to preserve the view. It must have extravasated or something and made its way through the abdomen and passed the diaphragm into the pleura. When he was extubated, he couldn't breathe. So...'

'I'm in the clear.'

He nodded but did not reply. Enough had been said.

That day I learned to wait and not to overreact. If you have done a good job, if it wasn't your fault, the truth will out.

1.10 Trust

Mrs. Banfield was septic, but we could not work out where the infection was coming from. Bacteria were circulating in her blood stream, but they must have come from somewhere. The usual list of sites – urine, lungs, gall bladder – had been investigated and had checked out. Her brain seemed fine, and there were no signs of meningitis. Next week, we might look at the heart valves, but for now, we knew what to do: start strong antibiotics and wait for them to improve the situation.

The antibiotic I was asked to prescribe was called gentamicin. I sighed. I hated it. In my view, it was dangerous, because if blood levels drifted up, beyond the 'therapeutic window', it could cause kidney failure or hearing loss. To prevent this, the junior doctor responsible had to check the levels and calculate the timing and the size of each dose. There were graphs and equations in the books to help, and although challenging, it was not beyond the abilities of an intelligent person. In Mrs. Banfield's case, there were additional risks: her kidneys were already failing because of multiple myeloma (bone marrow cancer), and even more worrying to me, it was Friday. I would not be there to make sure the blood test was taken at the right time, the result checked, the calculation made.

At 6 PM, I drew boxes on the drug chart to show when the doses were due, marked by asterisks and arrows to a comment – 'CHECK LEVEL'. I told the nurse in charge of the ward to keep an eye out, having confirmed that she was working on Saturday and Sunday. I called the doctor who would be covering the ward, but she had already gone home – unsurprisingly, as she had to be in 8 AM the next day. So I found the handover file and left clear instructions in an outlined box. There were already 15 other jobs for her to do on Saturday. I knew she would read this file on Saturday morning, and I knew her. She was conscientious.

On Saturday I wondered, should I call her? But I decided not to. There was a system for handing over tasks, and it worked. Her bleep would be going off incessantly, and the last thing she needed was me hassling her. I let it go, and by the evening was thoroughly distracted by whatever social engagement I had arranged, this being well before the time of children.

On Sunday, the same thought occurred – should I ring?

No. This was a kind of test. Was the system reliable enough to look after patients at the weekend? And was I able to let go? After all, I had a life outside the hospital. I had to be able to turn off.

Monday morning. I headed straight to Mrs. Banfield's ward. The curtains were drawn around her bed. I put my head through the gap and saw two doctors I did not recognise leaning over her. One of them, a consultant with grey hair, turned to look at me?

'Your patient?'

'Yes.'

'We're from ICU. She's in renal failure.'

'They were failing last week. The myeloma, probably.'

'That, and the gent.'

He held out the drug chart. My mind was too disturbed to focus on the little boxes that I had carefully drawn. I kept staring and saw that someone had prescribed 300 mg on Saturday. A big dose. The box that I had drawn, where the level should have been written, was empty. She had been re-dosed with no thought given to the residual concentration in her blood. The new dose of 300 mg must have sent her level way over the top. And now her kidneys, already struggling because of the sticky proteins being pushed out by her out of control bone marrow, had failed completely.

There was an investigation. I was asked to write an account of my actions. I had to say who I had handed the job over to. In her report, the other doctor described how the ED was very busy on Saturday night, forcing her to delegate the task of reviewing Mrs. Banfield's gentamicin prescription to a more junior doctor. He didn't understand about the levels properly. Forced to 'do something', anxious that the patient should not go without an antibiotic, he prescribed what he thought was a standard dose.

Mrs. Banfield improved with some haemofiltration. Then I moved to a different ward, and lost contact. I never knew if she survived her myeloma. I doubt it.

But I learned something. Don't leave things to chance. Don't worry too much about hassling people with phone calls. The stakes are too high. And if something is playing on your mind, deal with it. The stress of not doing something, and worrying about the consequences, will do more to spoil your weekend than the 10-minute interruption.

1.11 Paralysis

Four o'clock in the morning. I was called to see a patient in respiratory distress. Arriving at the door of the side room I saw a thin, immobile man on the verge of respiratory arrest. His body was misshapen, his legs flexed and wasted, his chest protuberant and barrel-shaped. There was an electric wheelchair in the corner of the room. The house officer, who had been struggling with him for 10 minutes, looked up.

'Spinal muscular atrophy. He's being treated for pneumonia, query aspiration[8].'

I lowered the back of the bed and with a bag and mask assisted his ventilation. A small bolus of adrenaline strengthened what had been a barely palpable pulse. He soon began to breathe more frequently and more deeply. He mumbled for the first time, and his eyes appeared to focus on those who were standing by his bed.

'He's probably good enough for some non-invasive ventilation...' I said, 'we might get away without intubating him. Can you carry on doing this for a minute, just squeezing the bag when he breathes... gently, I'm going to have a quick chat with his relatives.'

The relatives, his brother and sister, were waiting by the door. They had observed everything. I introduced myself, confirmed with them the nature of their brother's neurological condition and continued:

'The infection has progressed despite the antibiotics, and that, combined with his long-standing weakness, has restricted his breathing. The carbon dioxide has built up inside him and made him drowsy. He's a little better already, but he needs more help with his breathing.'

'Whatever it takes, doctor. Just get him better.'

'We will try, but I can't over-emphasise how unwell he is. He may need to go on a ventilator.' They nodded and gazed past me into the room. The nurse touched my arm and pointed to the door. I entered to see the patient looking pinker and stronger. He was grasping the house officer's hand, trying to push him away. The medical notes lay open on the bedside cabinet, where the house officer could read them.

'He's got cancer. Gastric cancer.'

'What?'

'It says here... these notes are so crap; it says he's recently had chemo.' I turned on my heels and left the room again.

'Excuse me. The notes indicate that your brother has been receiving treatment for stomach cancer.'

'Yes, he has.'

'When was this?'

'A few weeks ago. They said it was successful.'

'Has he had an operation?'

'No.'

'Is he due to have one?'

'I don't think so. They're just treating it with injections.'

'I'm sorry to be blunt... but this is very important... has he been told, or has he told you, that his cancer is incurable or terminal?'

'No. No, doctor.'

I paused, concerned that in the haste demanded by this situation, I appeared to be writing the patient off.

'Has he ever talked to you about what he would want if he fell seriously ill and needed intensive care, or a life support machine?'

'No.'

'He's never expressed an opinion about it?'

'About what?'

'About being kept alive on a ventilator.'

'No, never.'

The nurse stayed with the relatives. I joined the house officer in the side room and with a mobile internal phone arranged a bed on the respiratory ward. The patient was sitting up again now, still terribly distressed, but looking around. We arrived on the ward to find a non-invasive ventilator set up in readiness. I placed the mask over his nose and mouth. He grabbed my wrist, but I resisted the force and pressed hard to ensure an airtight seal. He cringed beneath the pressure of the plastic and shook his head again and again. The exaggerated bone structure of his emaciated face conveyed desperation and fear. It was impossible to fix the elastic straps behind his head. The relatives had followed us to the ward. His sister held his left hand.

'Let them put it on. You need it for your breathing. Let them do it. It won't be for long, will it, doctor?'

'No, not for long.'

'You see, it's just to get you over the infection.'

I tried again. He held his sister with his gaze for a few seconds, and then closed his eyes in submission. His head fell back onto the pillow, he became still, and the mask was at last secured.

'What now, doctor?'

'We'll have to see if this machine can do enough for him. If not, he will need to go on a ventilator.'

'Cancer. And not resected. There's something not right there,' replied the intensive care registrar when I called to warn him of the possible transfer.

'But the family tell me it's been treated successfully. I've got no other information. They are pushing for full active treatment. We're going to have to offer everything until we get the full story in the cold light of day. Even if we knew who his oncologist was, we could hardly call him at 4 in the morning.'

An hour and a half later, I called an anaesthetist. Mask ventilation had been unsuccessful. I watched as the patient was sedated, paralysed and intubated.

At midday, I passed through intensive care and asked the registrar how the patient was doing.

'We called his oncologist once the old notes had been retrieved from records... and he couldn't believe he'd been admitted to ICU. He's got inoperable, terminal cancer, a couple of months at most. We're pulling out once the relatives have had a chance to take it in. They're clueless.'

'I see. Sorry about all that.'

'Don't be... what can you do if the notes are incomplete? It's an impossible situation.'

It appears that I had little choice but to treat him aggressively. I have, however, omitted something, one brief interaction. It took place just after my conversation with the brother and sister concerning the patient's cancer. The nurse and the relatives were outside, leaving just the house officer and myself in the side room. In response to the fear that I had detected in the patient's eyes, I eased the rubber mask from his face and levelled my head in front of his.

'Do you want us to do this? Do you want us to help you?' I asked.

He could barely control his movements, but his eyes, ever articulate, spoke volumes. And in addition, I detected, as I think the house officer did, a slow, controlled shake of the head. His answer was 'No'.

A disastrous situation. The last 48 hours of a terminally ill man's life were transformed into a demonstration of medicine's resuscitative prowess: ventilators, central lines, inotropes, discomfort combined with powerlessness... the last being a price worth paying if the underlying disease process is reversible, and the life regained worth living. Not so in this case. So why did it happen?

It would not have developed were it not for the inefficient transfer of information. The team that admitted this patient had no idea of the severity of his disease. In the absence of his old notes, their only source of information was the family, and they seemed genuinely to believe that his cancer had been treated 'successfully'. Either he had misunderstood the words of his oncologist, or perhaps – and this is most likely – the patient had given them a sanitised version. The notes being incomplete (comprising only the casualty card and two sheets of A4 paper on which the findings and decisions made during two ward rounds had been made), there was no clue as to the extent of the patient's knowledge, nor an indication of his wishes should he become unwell.

More importantly, why did I ignore the patient's wish to be left to die? In essence, I decided that action would be easier to defend than inaction, even if, in my view, positive action was not in the patient's best interests. The factors that swayed this decision were the relatives' obvious desire that their 'successfully' treated brother 'get better', and the reflex that is trained into doctors to *do something* when presented with a patient on the verge of death. Wilting against these powerful forces for action stood my *perception* that the patient did not want to be 'saved'.

He could not talk. He could only look at me in an accusatory manner and shake his head. I might easily (and reasonably, to my peers) have dismissed the patient as not competent to make such a decision, given his shocked state. But he was competent, and his opinion was clear. Nevertheless, I could not bring myself to stand before the relatives and say: 'He does not want to be put through all this.'

'How do you know? Has he told you?' they would reply.

'Not exactly, but I'm sure it's what he wants. I can see it in his eyes.'

This scenario, which concerns the question of life sustaining treatment in the context of uncertainty is one that is commonly met on the wards, especially out of hours, when the doctors on call are summoned to patients about whom they have no knowledge. The element in this particular case, which drives us to dissect the motives behind the decisions we make, is the shake of the head. Subjective, brief, easily erased by a mind craving simplicity and comfort… it immediately juxtaposed what the patient *wanted* with what I knew I *had* to do.

What my reaction to this mute signal tells us is that, however strong our conviction that treatment is not in a patient's best interests, we will compromise in the face of pressure from relatives, or in a situation where death is likely to result from our lack of action. We treat, for that is what doctors do, and we are unlikely to be criticised for it. It is this fear of criticism, be it professional, legal or merely vociferous, that is thus revealed as a prime motivator when difficult decisions are contemplated.

Clinical decisions are therefore seen to be modulated by professional and legal paranoia. They are scrutinised in the light of the question: 'How will this make me look?' Usually, the doctor's best interests coincide with the patient's, but this is not always so, and was probably not so in the case described here. The decision to treat this patient was based on *my* concerns about *my* situation. It would have taken an exceptionally brave, slightly naïve doctor to have acted otherwise.

This case changed me. It made an indelible mark, a classic 'necessary scar'. Since then I have always tried to explore patients' desires and goals near the end of life. Sometimes a few words is all you need to hear. 'Leave me alone.' 'Don't put me on a machine.' Better the hard conversation now, than the dreadful sense of emergency that took over this man's final hours.

1.12 Zone

A rare visit to the ED. As a consultant, I have become accustomed to having my patients filtered by teams of admitting teams and transferred to a specialist ward. Now things have changed. Coronavirus has turned everything upside-down. There is no more hiding in my silo. Here I am, 11 o'clock at night, seeing patients fresh off the street, straight off the ED trainee's bat. She saw Mr Kafkasis, quickly ascertained that he needed to be admitted and referred him along to me, the medical consultant.

I see Mr Kafkasis in the company of a trainee; he has three or four years of experience. He is keen and he has expressed an interest in my specialty. Good lad!

Even better, the patient has liver disease. I examine him, and demonstrate a couple of signs to educate the trainee (he nods appreciatively, but he has seen them before; perhaps he humours me). We analyse the blood tests together; our heads close over the COW (computer-on-wheels). The liver looks alright, on paper, but we know there is a major problem. Mr Kafkasis's abdomen has filled with fluid, approximately 12 litres, I reckon (actually, I whisper, I'm quite well known for the accuracy of my estimates).

The trainee points out that the patient is anaemic. I nod in agreement. It's no surprise. Cirrhosis does that. His red cells are reduced in size, which is a little atypical, but not inconsistent. Small red cells usually mean there is iron deficiency, which in turn means internal bleeding. Mr Kafkasis flatly denies seeing any blood, from either end, but part of my plan is to arrange an endoscopy into his stomach. That should answer the question. The main issues are to do with his liver: he needs a whole new batch of blood tests (I reel them off, confidently; this is my area after all, my comfort zone), a scan, a sample of abdominal fluid needs to be drawn off and analysed... then, assuming no infection, he can have those 12 litres drained tomorrow.

I am not running the ward next day, so Mr Kafkasis is seen by a colleague. A week later, I ask after him over coffee, as I like to know what comes of my decisions. Was I right, does he have schistosomiasis?[9] It is too early to know; the blood test must have be sent away. What did the endoscopy show? Nothing really, we gave him some blood and an iron infusion because of the anaemia, and he's due to go home. The anaemia is odd, we'll have to look into it further, says my colleague. I nod absently. It doesn't seem that relevant to me.

Three weeks later, the same colleague comes into my office.

'You remember Mr Kafkasis?'

'Of course. That schisto result back yet?'

'No. But he's got rectal cancer.'

I swivel my chair around to face her squarely. 'What?'

'We arranged a colonoscopy, because of the anaemia, and it was scheduled for this morning. Mike did it. But he felt the cancer at rectal examination before he put the 'scope in.'

'He's taken biopsies.'

'Yes, he could get the 'scope past the tumour. He took photos. It's definitely a cancer.'

I pause. Is she thinking what I'm thinking? I say it first;

'He never had a rectal exam, did he? Not in ED, not on the ward.'

'No.' She talks over the omission, my omission, by describing how she has arranged an MRI scan and referred to the surgeons. Then she leaves me.

It was my job to have ensured that the rectal exam was performed. Not necessarily by me, but by the trainee, or by the team next day. Because that's what you do when examining patients with anaemia, especially if the red cells are small. That's what you do.

But I did not make it happen, because I was luxuriating in my comfort zone, playing the teacher, focusing on the things that came easily to me.

1.13 Prison

There is a new email in my inbox:

> A patient well known to you, Gary Folkestone, was admitted to ICU overnight; please can you review on the ward round? Septic, decompensated liver failure.

Oh yes, I remember the man. He was on my ward two weeks ago, bright yellow with jaundice, swollen in the face and the legs. An alcoholic, a 'recidivist' as we used to say; an archaic term meaning 'a convicted criminal who reoffends, especially repeatedly' or, in earlier more religious times, a catholic who keeps sinning. A pejorative term, surely, but accepted shorthand in my world.

Gary didn't want to be in hospital. He had been scooped off the street by paramedics in a state of inebriation, but as soon as he came around, he began to fight to leave. He was transferred to my ward, and I assessed him. It was clear that his liver had stopped working, poisoned by vodka (Gary's favoured drink) over many years. I could feel its swollen edge and smell the sweet foetor of organ failure on his breath. On that day, he was mentally brighter, having received treatment overnight.

'I want to go,' he said.

'Well, hang on,' I replied. 'We need some more time to get you better.'

'I'm fine.'

'You're not fine. Have you looked in a mirror? You're bright yellow.'

'I feel better.'

'That's because you've been given fluids and vitamins and something to help the toxins that were building up in the brain. But you are still in danger.'

'I've got to go.'

'Why?'

'I'm meeting somebody.'

'They'll understand, Gary. Let's just agree on today, shall we? See how today goes. You will stay, won't you?'

'No. I'm going. I've already called my mate; he's picking me up during his lunch hour.'

'We can't...look, Gary, if you go home there's a good chance your liver will finally stop and you'll be brought back in a coma, or with bleeding. You'll be back to square one.'

'That's not going to happen. Look, Doctor, I've been very reasonable...I've stayed in overnight...'

And so it starts. The suggestion, that we, the doctors and nurses, have somehow imposed this visit to the hospital on him.

'...I let them take blood last night, let them put this cannula in... I've got people I need to see, things to do...'

As though the decisions we made were to inconvenience him.

'Those things were done to save your life. You were in a coma when you came in.'

'I'm grateful, doctor. But I'm going. Today.'

What next? What do I say?

I have heard all the following categories of response in this type of situation. Some sound wrong, but are understandable; some are morally right but medically unsafe. Which did I choose?

'This is a hospital, not a prison...' The classic riposte. It's true, of course; treatment is entirely voluntary, and a patient, having been informed about the risks, has the perfect right to walk away. To me, this response represents a complete breakdown of the physician–patient relationship. It is a surrender, to the complexity of the challenge. You might as well say what you're thinking, which is 'Fine, I'm DONE with you!'

How does this conversation end? Often, with this – 'But you will need to sign a self-discharge form.' This may crystallise, in the mind of the patient, the fact that responsibility for what happens to them from that point on is all theirs. It is a form of brinkmanship, watching to see if they change their mind as they write their name. Brinkmanship really has no place in good medicine.

'We'll let you go... but you must understand, if you do deteriorate, your bed will be gone, you'll need to call an ambulance and come to A and E...' The blackmail. By describing how difficult it will be to re-engage with the hospital, you hope to dissuade him. You avoid invoking the emotional angle, emphasising how disappointed you are that all the 'hard work will be undone', but the loss of 'the bed' signifies this. The bed is the symbol of the care that they have received, and by losing it to another patient, they sacrifice the therapeutic bond that duty and need forged in you.

Gary's departure will be semi-condoned, so as not to require a self-discharge letter. But this is risky, from the point of view of the doctors, for if Gary does collapse and die on the high street, the medical team will have no documentation with which to defend themselves. By maintaining a relationship, they open themselves up to criticism.

'I understand, Gary, I'd want to go if I were in your position. But give us another 24, 48 hours...please. That's all we need. Then we'll get you home, I promise.' The bargain. A false one at that, because you have no idea what the next day or two will hold. He may require another chest drain, or worse, transfer to a cardio-thoracic unit... it's a lie (albeit well intentioned) to promise anything in medicine. You have paid for his compliance by making a commitment that you may not be able to fulfil. The push back, in two days, may be all the more intense.

'I understand, Gary, I'd want to go if I were in your position. Let's see what we can work out.' And you go on to explore a true compromise. He goes home, but you arrange for him to come up to the ward every day for a quick check over; or for the SHO to call him, to make sure he is still breathing well; or for the General Practitioner (GP) to do the same. A truly personalised approach. It sounds like good medicine – it takes into account his specific concerns, his anxiety to get back to work, his need for freedom!

But is it realistic? By making these arrangements, you create extra work and unusual demands on your team, or the GP. Gary either needs to be monitored or he does not; and if he does, he needs to be in hospital. It's as simple as that. What sounds and feels reasonable may actually be unreasonable, even if it does maintain the therapeutic relationship.

'I understand that you need to leave. But let's think about this…let's put it into perspective.' Thus speaks the philosopher. You go on to explain, 'Gary, if you don't make a full recovery from this, you could be in and out of hospital for weeks, months. If you can just spend some time focusing on your health now, even if it takes longer than you'd like, you can get better properly and avoid longer-term problems. Then, a year from now, looking back on this time, it will be just a blip…you'll be back at work, with it all behind you.' Such subtle mind-tricks can work, because they are, in fairness, reasonable. Patients who cannot accept their ill health, who continuously resist management plans that will entail longer periods of hospitalisation, might benefit from the odd dose of perspective. The danger, from the doctor's point of view, is that of sounding patronising. After all, it's not you who are away from work and family for weeks on end. The problem with this approach is that it doesn't change a thing, materially.

Finally, there is the approach that fewer doctors, in busy wards, confronted by aggression or apparent ingratitude, will take; that of sitting down, ignoring the rush of oncoming clinical traffic, and exploring what it is, really, that troubles the patient. For there is bound to be a source of stress, be it financial, inter-personal or domestic that can be identified and addressed. Perhaps it's an addiction; perhaps it's their turn to look after the kids this weekend. To find out what it is requires an ability to ignore the simmering anger, and to understand the emotional heat created when illness afflicts younger generations who are used to running their own lives quite satisfactorily in normal circumstances. A tall order, that only the most disciplined can succeed in – and on a good day at that.

I looked at Gary. We had already spent 20 minutes at his bedside. There was no persuading him. The electronic record showed that he had been admitted 20 times or more over the last 18 months. The alcohol support team could make no headway with him. Whatever his history, whatever misfortune had befallen him earlier in life, however poor the role models were in his household as a youth, I was not going to succeed in turning him around. Gary knew what he wanted. He had the mental capacity to make his own decisions. I reverted to cliché:

'Well, Gary, this is a hospital, not a prison…'

And off he walked.

I stood over him in the ICU. Soft, transparent pads covered his closed eyes to protect them. A breathing tube rested on the dirty, irregular teeth of his lower jaw. The jaundice was worse than before. There was a bruise on one cheek. Numerous infusion units pumped drugs into his vein to maintain blood pressure, fight infection and keep him asleep so that he did not fight the ventilator. His nurse summarised the situation for me,

'The consultant just came round. She wanted to discuss it with you, but she's thinking of setting some limits of care as he's deteriorating despite high dose norad.

She doesn't really want to filter him, given the state of his liver... not being a transplant candidate.'

I nodded. Yes, I agreed. Gary wasn't making it out of here. His liver was gone now. He was dying.

I left the ICU and paused by a window. I replayed our final conversation. I *could* have persuaded him to stay. It would have meant slowing down, taking a seat by his bed and unwrapping his motives. But I didn't give him the time. And he had annoyed me, making it sound like we had *made* him come in, tortured him with blood tests, pinned him to the bed... It wasn't the doctors who destroyed his liver; it was him. His actions. But I'm a liver specialist. I know the scientific literature. The 'social determinants of health' have been well described. His socio-economic background, his upbringing, his underlying addictive personality, his need to escape the daily grind of life in vodka's misty glaze, combined perfectly to guarantee his alcoholism and a premature death.

But this is not a prison, and he was clear.

He wanted to leave, and I let him.

1.14 Burn

We are not running late exactly, but it is already 10.30 and we have not started the first of two morning cases yet. The patient requires deep sedation, and the anaesthetist has never met her before. He has lots of questions. I leave the room, so as not to be seen to be pressurising him. They are a very 'safe' lot, these anaesthetists. Lots of checks, nothing left to chance. Frustrating, when you are waiting to start surgery or a procedure, but, so slow...

I return, and – hooray! – she is asleep. She has not been given paralysing drugs, so she can breathe for herself. But now I am embarrassed, because I wasn't there to go through the checklist while the patient was still conscious. The list of questions is not long – 10 or so – but some of them do require the patient's input. Such as: Do you have any allergies? Do you have any breathing problems? The anaesthetist would have picked these things up though. I run through the questions. Name check – a nurse confirms the patient's identity by examining the wristband. Allergies? – the anaesthetist shakes his head. I knew he'd check. Anti-coagulants or blood thinners – no, says the nurse who checked the drug history. Pacemaker or implant? – the anaesthetist looks blank; not his area (I disagree, but he isn't looking interested). She is only 50 and is not likely to have a heart problem. I feel the skin across the top of the chest; there is no telltale bump. Breathing problems? – well, she's on a ventilator, no need to worry about that. Diabetes – no. Dentures – no. Equipment needed available – yes. Done. I sign it and prepare to start the procedure.

Early on in the procedure, I ask my assistant to connect the diathermy, because I need to make a small incision internally. My right foot depresses the yellow pedal on the floor, and the cut is nicely made, and bloodless. But the patient has moved. Her back is arching! Her face is stretched with pain, despite the deep sedation.

'What's that?' I ask.

The anaesthetist looks worried. They say anaesthetics is 99% boredom and 1% sheer terror. She is writhing on the bed. I am clueless. I remove the instrument I was using. The anaesthetist says,

'Let's wake her up. We need to know what's happening, maybe it's a seizure.' He is standing over her head looking into her eyes, testing the pupils for reaction to light.

Then one of the nurses who was helping me with the equipment says,

'Hang on, she said something about her back outside... what was it...'

I wait. 'Yes... what?'

'She said she had a pain moderator, modulator, something... in her back...'

Oh God. She's got a spinal stimulator, and I passed electric current through her body. It will have travelled along the wires and cooked her spinal cord... oh God...

I am sorry. Sorry to you, the reader. This did not happen.

    « Rewind «
    > Play >

We are not running late exactly, but it is already 10.30 and we have not started the first of two morning cases yet. The patient requires deep sedation, and the anaesthetist has never met her before. He has lots of questions. I leave the room, so as not to be seen to be pressurising him. They are a very 'safe' lot, these anaesthetists. Lots of checks, nothing left to chance. Frustrating, when you are waiting to start surgery or a procedure, but, so slow...

I approach the anaesthetist.

'Sorry, before you put her to sleep we just need to do our checklist.'

'Go for it.'

The list of questions is not long – ten or so – but some of them do require the patient's input. Such as: Name check – she repeats it for the umpteenth time. Do you have any allergies? She shakes her head. Do you have any breathing problems? 'Not that I know of.' Any anti-coagulants or blood thinners – 'No.' Pacemaker or implant? – 'No... hang on, I've got a paraspinal stimulator for chronic pain. Does that count.?' 'It most definitely does,' I reply. 'We can't use any electricity inside, but we can find ways around that.' Breathing problems? – well, she's on a ventilator, no need to worry about that. Diabetes – no. Dentures – no. Equipment needed available – yes. Done. I sign it and prepare to start the procedure.

It goes well, and she is home by tea-time.

Why put you through the fictional drama? Because when she told me about the spinal stimulator, I could not believe that she had got this far without anyone noticing it or mentioning it. It was the checklist that gave her time to recall that there *was* something embedded under the skin... something that she should mention to me. I was five minutes away from pressing the pedal and using electricity. Four years ago, before we brought checklists into our routine, I would probably have proceeded... and she may have ended up paralysed. Another medical accident. I could not stop myself visualising what might have happened if the correct question had not been asked. I scared myself with the vision of her paralysis and created an artificial scar in my psyche. It has motivated me to comply with the checklist. It has worked.

'You like safety, don't you?' somebody once asked me. I nodded. Who doesn't? But that does not mean I embrace every 'safe' innovation. Yes, I support them, if they are well evidenced. I champion them. But deep down... sometimes I think, *God, this just makes my life harder.* That was my initial reaction to checklists.

The case for them has been made so well. Atul Gawande eulogised them in a long *New Yorker* article (2.12.2007), the NHS adopted them, airlines have relied on them for decades (watch how pilot Chesley Sullenberger reaches across for one as soon as his engines lose power in Clint Eastwood's film *Sully*, 2016). They work. Yet, doctors don't like them. They are an effort, an obstacle, an apparently petty imposition. I know it's the right patient! I know they're not on warfarin! I know what equipment we need to do the procedure. It's all so obvious. Yet, now and again, something goes wrong. Never Events occur. The wrong patient is operated on, the wrong tooth or kidney is removed, or an allergy is missed and a drug that is dangerous to them is injected. Checklists reduce these events, so what's the problem?

My experience with checklists has been interesting. I am a proponent, a kind of champion, yet even now, after my near-miss, I often huff and puff as, on the brink of putting an endoscope down, the wretched piece of paper is waved at me.

The process of completing the particular checklist that we have developed takes a minute at most. It requires standing still (a problem when you're in a hurry), focusing the team's attention on the responses (for what is the point of the patient telling me they are allergic to something if no one else in the room is aware?) and communicating with the patient (a problem for some, especially when in a hurry).

Perhaps it's this need to pause and be still that frustrates doctors and surgeons. We, they, like to keep moving, to flow through the tasks, to get to the nitty gritty (the technique, the findings, the pathology, the treatment) as soon as possible. It is this habit that is so difficult to break. It is a mind-set. And it reveals something about our approach to our surgical lists. They are our lists. They have our names on them. Their character – relaxed, rushed, efficient, friendly, spikey, miserable – stems from our own behaviour and the clinical leads in the room. The checklist is an obstacle to our progress through the day and to a successful outcome. With this mind-set, the fact that it is the patient's procedure can be forgotten; forgotten also the fact that around the surgeon buzzes a team of highly assistants without whom the procedure could not take place. The checklist is the best – probably only – way to ensure that for a moment, everyone is focused on that patient, and the last opportunity to identify possible harm is heeded.

Gradually, slowly, the checklist should become natural, and depending on your psychology, you feel that something is missing without it. We used not to clean our hands before and after every patient contact; now, if I haven't, I feel kind of tainted, as though there is something on my skin that hasn't been taken off. They are clean, of course, but the habit has become so ingrained my mind insists on the slap of antiseptic foam before moving on. In the same way, the checklist should become a door through which your mind insists on moving before embarking on the procedure.

I'm not sure I'm at that stage yet. If there are distractions, or if I am running very late, the checklist can be overlooked, until a colleague holds it up and pulls me back. I know that if harm does occur in relation to a surgical procedure, the absence of a checklist looks bad. Completed correctly, it serves to protect you, as the surgeon. It demonstrates that care was taken, and thought given to the patient as an individual, not as a 'procedure'.

Most doctors and nurses are already converted. But the checklist mentality remains a change, and a challenge. As Gawande[10] says, comparing the flair and fluidity with which surgeons like to move through their lists with the early astronauts from *The Right Stuff*,

> ...the prospect [of checklists] pushes against the traditional culture of medicine, with its central belief that in situations of high risk and complexity what you want is a kind of expert audacity — the right stuff, again. Checklists and standard operating procedures feel like exactly the opposite, and that's what rankles many people.

Expert audacity vs regimentation, again in Gawande's words. This points to the same psychology I explored above. The audacity, the flair, the speed, all relate to the surgeon.

But it's the patient's procedure.

2

Words: Failures in Communication

Medicine is as much about communication as it is about using your hands or making decisions. The wrong words can do more harm than an incorrect prescription. Words – the way they are delivered and the feelings they generate – are what patients remember. Communication skills are hard to teach. In medical school, it is soon clear who can and can't communicate, and as a new doctor on the wards of my first hospital, I remember grimacing when particularly inept consultants gave bad news from on high, moving on before the dust and rubble raised by their verbal bombshells had begun to settle. For me, learning how to communicate well largely became a process of negative role modelling – avoiding the methods of the notably bad. But as the scenes that follow demonstrate, I am still no expert.

2.1 Limit

The first opportunity I had to break bad news was three months after I had left medical school. A middle-aged man had collapsed and lay unconscious behind a curtain. A brain scan showed that he had suffered a haemorrhagic stroke; a blood vessel in his brain had burst open, leading to a clot to form within the delicate tissue. I was ready to face his family, and my registrar was happy to let me do it. She had seen me on the wards, and felt agreed that it was time.

We entered a specially furnished family room; the walls were pastel peach and an innocuous landscape painting had been hung. A box of tissues lay at an angle on the coffee table, one tissue half-pulled.

I told them what had happened in clear, honest terms. The wife took it calmly and had no specific questions. The son however was far more focused. He wanted to know what proportion of patients woke up, if surgery was being considered, what sort of surgery could be done and how many recovered after surgery. He asked about what medications we were giving and if there was a bed available in the city's neurosurgical unit. I parried each question with a generalisation or non-verifiable fact based on the scanty knowledge of neurosurgery I had acquired during my studies. My pride insisted that I fulfil the role that I had assigned myself - the all-knowing doctor. The son was becoming frustrating, looking up at the ceiling, exuding exasperation. I half-expected him to turn to his mother and say, 'This is just a kid; he doesn't know shit!'. Then I came clean.

'I'm sorry, but I'm not an expert. I can tell you what has happened, and what we need to do, for now. We have sent his brain scan across to the neurosurgeon on call, but it is such a specialised area I can't predict what they will say. I can't say what his chances of recovery are. It's too early. But I know this is terribly serious. He is still

DOI: 10.1201/9781003189824-2

unconscious, and that is a very worrying sign. You should prepare for the worst. I'm sorry.'

The son appeared to relax, and his frame loosened on the bland yellow sofa. The wife smiled at me, perhaps a little knowingly, as though she had known the truth all along. I was a messenger, not a bad one, but not the decision maker. I was not in charge of her husband's case.

I left the family room gladly. And I vowed never to enter one again without knowing *everything* about the condition of the patient I was planning to discuss.

2.2 Proximity

Years later, I contemplated another bad news conversation. I knew exactly what the diagnosis was, I could speak confidently about the possible treatments, I had an onward plan prepared to allow some positive focus, a constructive approach. He's bound to ask about prognosis, I thought, but I'll have to deflect that…it's too early to get into numbers. He's going to need to see an oncologist. This is just the first hurdle – breaking the bad news. He has an inkling, I know, but we haven't talked about it openly. I know how to do this.

There will be a quiet, private room. There will be two seats, for him and his partner. I'm going to switch off my phone. The diary is clear for an hour; we can talk for as long as necessary. I've done it before; I've seen worse. It's not exactly routine, but it's part of the job.

He's not much older than me. He shouldn't have something this serious. I think he's got young children. Last time I saw him he was on his own, on the ward. We drew some fluid and sent it off for analysis. This is a follow-up appointment, arranged urgently after the report landed on my desk. I did mention some possibilities at the time, as I was suspicious even at that early stage. I have no idea if he shared his fears with his partner. She's coming with him though.

What does he need from me? He's a fairly matter-of-fact man, he just wants to get to the facts. And that's how I'm going to be. I've got the facts, but I haven't got the whole story. I can't tell him how long he's got. But I can provide a clear interpretation of the facts that I do have. I've done it many times.

That I'm thinking so much about this means something. I tell people every week that they have potentially lethal diseases, but this one is bugging me. I think it's because he and I are similar. We're at similar stages in our different careers; we both have young families. Am I nervous because I fear for myself when I see him? Am I worried that his misfortune will contaminate me? What is going on if *my* response to *his* illness is concern for *my* own future? If bad luck was contagious, I'd be dead by now.

It's different with the elderly; serious illness is an almost inevitable part of ageing. And they tend to take it with little expressed emotion. What was it I read the other day? *'He had reached an age where death no longer has the quality of ghastly surprise…' The Great Gatsby*. A book about young people. This man is being halted in his prime. I find myself thinking about how I would react if it was me. I'm thinking about it too much, that's the problem.

I am walking to the clinic. It's quiet in the department as I arranged to use a room over the lunch hour. They haven't arrived yet. I go through the notes, but there is no new information. A nurse opens the door and tells me he has arrived. He enters with his partner; they take their seats.

'How are you?' It's an irrelevant question, a needless pleasantry.

'Okay. Have you got the results?'

'Yes. There are abnormal cells in the fluid. Cancer cells.' His partner juts forward. 'You mean it's cancer?'

'Yes.' Straight facts, that's what they need.

I look at him. He is sweating. He is no longer receptive to my words.

His phone vibrates. In a matter-of-fact way, as is his manner, he pulls it out of his jacket pocket to read the text. I think he's consciously carrying on as normal. I glance at his phone and see the image that he has saved to his home screen. Two children. I am rocked by the sudden realisation that he is not going to see them grow up. I stutter. I am very uncomfortable. The professionalism, the experience, the constructive momentum that I hoped would facilitate this consultation, have faded to nothing. I lose my way repeatedly, failing to find a secure path between his need for information and her evolving horror.

10 minutes later, they leave. I have laid out the short-term plan, forced it onto the table, and I have avoided the big question about prognosis. But it didn't go well. I know it didn't go well. How could it, really? But my 'performance' was not right. For a few moments, I was swimming in the murky waters of that couple's emotional pain, and I was not doing my job. Perhaps they noticed. She did, I'm pretty sure.

Empathy is vital in the practice of medicine. It involves understanding a patient's condition from their perspective. But it lies on a spectrum, with 'detached concern' at one end, and over-identification at the other. In this instance I over-identified. Next time I would play it cool. Think less. Feel less. Stay professional.

A year later, I had moved too far along that spectrum.

2.3 Radius

I explained to Sandra and her family that the liver was packed with cancer. The cause for the pain she had been experiencing for the last three weeks was now clear. There was no cure. The primary source was a mystery; it was an 'unknown primary'. Family members occupied the bedside spaces; three were seated, but a young man – the son – stood. He had declined a chair. He looked down intensely, and when I had said my piece he asked sensible questions about discharge arrangements and follow-up appointments. It was he, I felt, who would organise things and communicate to the wider family. The situation was challenging for me, but not unusual or especially complex from a purely medical point of view. Such conversations are required on a weekly basis. Sandra was sitting up, passive but fully aware, despite a recent dose of morphine. She took it all in but would probably rely on those around her to process most of the information.

I finished, said goodbye and left the ward. The sadness of the situation melted away as I progressed along the corridor. There were other things on my mind, numerous tasks of a different nature. The family? They were behind the curtains – staring, crying, wondering.

A colleague approached. He had just returned from holiday. I stopped. He told me a story; one of his children said something hilarious to a flight attendant on the way home. I laughed out loud, letting out a snort of amusement. 'You are *kidding*!' A man brushed past me on his way to the stairwell, mobile phone in hand. The son! He looked round and recognised me, the doctor who just a few minutes ago described in measured, soft tones how his mother would soon die. My mouth was still open, genuine mirth colouring my face. His expression was neutral, and he turned away to push the door open. I regained my composure.

I was embarrassed.

I wondered – how wide is the radius of grief within which you should maintain the dignity of one who has just communicated a death sentence? When is it appropriate to relax and be yourself again? Should one be embarrassed to accept that life goes on for those unaffected by illness? Just around the corner, joy visits the hospital daily in the labour ward. For every death, a new arrival. Sometimes you see happy grandparents waiting with balloons or flowers in the same corridor as commiserating relatives who have received bad news.

Yet, yet... I wished he hadn't caught me at that moment, laughing so freely. The sympathy I displayed must have been skin deep; the performance, so empathic, was just a cameo. Was the son offended?

Next time I would put a greater distance between myself and the epicentre of grief.

2.4 Comfort

In Abraham Verghese's book *Cutting for Stone* (Vintage, 2009), the protagonist, a young doctor called Marion, seeks out his estranged father who has become a famous, and rather forbidding, liver transplant surgeon in Boston, MA. Unseen, Marion sneaks into a case conference. His father asks the audience of trainees,

'What treatment in an emergency is administered by ear?'

Marion knows the answer, having heard it from his father's lips as a child in his native Ethiopia. After a few moments, Marion puts his hand up.

'Words of comfort.'

Reassurance, a powerful tool. Perhaps too powerful.

A young patient, Sarah, well known to me through multiple previous visits, was admitted to the hospital once again. She had become severely jaundiced and the cause, as usual, was heavy drinking. Just a month ago, she had spent three weeks in hospital being fed via a nasal tube and receiving steroid tablets to calm down the dangerous inflammation in her liver. This time Sarah was even more unwell. Her arms and legs were thin, her abdomen was swollen and she was confused. But, as before, after a few days her strength began to return, and the jaundice improved. Her family came in. They tried to convince her to stay at home with them in order to watch over her, but she preferred to live in a shared house, with her friends, friends who supplied her with alcohol.

As I left one night, I saw Sarah's sister walk onto the ward. 'Pretty stable.' I told her. We knew that she was unlikely to survive more than six months, given the gradual decline in her liver function, but the time that she spent outside the hospital was satisfactory to her, and not without pleasure, or freedom. We had made every effort to help her recover from alcoholism, but to no avail.

As I drove in one morning, I received a phone call to say that Sarah had vomited two pints of blood on the ward. I parked the car and rushed in, knowing that she would need to be admitted to the ICU for resuscitation and an emergency endoscopy. She lay on her side, a puddle of congealing blood extending from her head to her chest on the bed sheet. The floor was sticky with it. She was groaning, but still conscious, fully aware of what was going on. The curtains had been pulled around all the other patients' beds so that they did not have to witness this terrible scene.

Within 15 minutes, she had been transferred to the ICU, and preparations were made to sedate and intubate her. This would allow me to perform an endoscopy without her struggling and moving around. I stood over her and she looked up. I explained what we were planning to do. She said, 'Doctor, just tell me I'm going to wake up from this.' I hesitated and said, 'Yes, we should be able to stop the bleeding and stabilise you; you should be awake in a couple of days.' An oxygen mask was put over her face, and the first sedative was administered.

I had lied to her. I knew her liver was probably not strong enough to sustain her through this massive haemorrhage. Privately, I gave her a 10 to 20% chance, at most, of pulling through. A large enough chance to justify aggressive treatment, especially for such a young patient, but a long shot. As the anaesthetist began to insert the endotracheal tube, a dark fountain rose up from her mouth and poured onto the already sodden pillow. Twin rivulets of blood fell from her nostrils. Her hair was matted with it.

When I passed the endoscope into her oesophagus, all I could see was red. I then inserted a balloon into the stomach to squeeze the engorged vessels from below, but her blood had become too thin and she continued to bleed. I tensed the balloon as much as possible, but over the next two hours, she lost more blood and her heart began to fail. The family arrived and I spoke with them. Death was now certain. She died half an hour later. It was no surprise – not to me, not to the nurses, not to the other consultants who looked after her in the past. But I could not forget that one of her last human interactions was with me, when I gave her reassurance that she would survive. I wonder if, as the sedatives kicked in, and the sound and the meaning of my words drifted across her darkening mind, they offered any comfort at all.

What should I do next time? Offer no comfort at all? Use bland words framed with caveats? 'I do believe you can make it through this... though bear in mind the data indicate a three-month survival of 27%...' The question is, did my words help in the moment? Did Sarah fall into unconsciousness believing that she would ascend again, to see her loved ones? Did my false words act like an opiate? A final palliative?

I will never know, because she is dead.

2.5 Cruel

I am not afraid to deliver hard news. That was my agenda on this occasion. Mr Chandra, an elderly and slightly overweight Asian man with a fatty, scarred liver, had been in and out of the hospital several times, his cognitive and physical status fluctuating due to the underlying condition. There was no cure. They walked into the clinic, husband and wife, I got into it quickly,

'So... the last few months, I've noticed, you've got weaker every time you've come in. The complications have been more difficult to get over. At home... you're not getting out...'

He said nothing. Perhaps today was an off day, mentally.

'So, we need to think about the future. What should we do next time you come in. And if you get *really* ill, an infection, or...'

His wife shifted in her seat.

I went on, using words I have used many times. About how there was only so much we could do if he deteriorated. About the possibility of spending his last days or weeks at home, if it looked like he might be dying. About things that might happen suddenly. Uncomfortable considerations, but necessary.

'But, doctor, he's doing OK really, isn't he?'

What? Where was this coming from? I moved my gaze from the patient to his wife. She was winking at me. A classic, conspiratorial wink. No, I would not have this....

'Well, it's important that we are very clear, and honest, about what we have seen over the last year. It's been a downward trend...'

'But now he's stable, isn't he? He's alright.'

I looked at him. He was looking at her.

'Don't want to hear any bad news, do we?' she said.

'No. No. There's enough to worry about in the world...' he replied, laughing quietly.

I paused. The signals were clear. This was not the time to push it. So, I changed tack.

'Well,' I continued, 'To be fair, you haven't been in for two months now. The new drug we gave you for the confusion seems to be working. And...' I turned to the computer, 'Looking at your numbers, your blood tests, there hasn't been much change there either. So yes, pretty stable!' I was getting into it now. The conspiracy of optimism. He needed this – this gentle fiction.

We wrapped things up. I had achieved nothing definite in terms of anticipating how to handle future crises. We would have to see how it went. So much for my agenda. Perhaps that was the problem, developing an agenda in isolation.

'Back in two months then?' I suggested, 'Unless you have to come in earlier.'

They walked out. There would be another time. Or, more likely, the hard truths, although fully understood, would remain unsaid until the very end.

There are other times when to tell the truth would appear cruel. After a week in hospital, Mrs. Greening, in her late 80s, had failed to improve from a chest infection. Her frailty meant that her chances of making it out of hospital were shrinking. We were duty-bound to discuss resuscitation. I knew what I thought: there was no way it would work. Before we entered the bay, I asked the team what they thought – all agreed. Was that their true opinion, or were they just following my lead? All one can do is ask. I looked to the senior nurse. She agreed too. It was not a difficult decision, medically. 'By the way,' said the nurse, 'It's her birthday.'

I approached the bed space. Mrs. Greening was drowsy, but a hand on the shoulder and gentle rock caused her to wake. She had all her mental faculties, full 'capacity', as we say. I knew already that there were no family members living nearby. I started in the usual way, with a brief examination and review of the latest blood tests. Then I prepared to deliver my line – 'I thought we should talk about what might happen if you get worse... if your breathing or your heart deteriorates... there's a chance that your heart could stop suddenly... it's called a cardiac arrest...'

Her thin arm lay outside the sheet, and I glanced at the name band. The date and the month... today. There were no cards, no flowers. I paused. Was she even aware? 'It's your birthday,' I said. 'Yes,' she replied, in a neutral tone. It had no significance for her. Birthdays are only as special as the people around you.

Images of her as a young girl waking up in a state of excitement, 80 years ago, entered my mind. The juxtaposition between youthful health, optimism, a life not yet lived, and present reality... was stark. My words, formally raising the prospect of death, would symbolise the end of the dreams and ambitions she had nurtured. Perhaps most were fulfilled. I did not know.

'Well, happy birthday anyway,' I muttered. She smiled weakly. We moved to the next patient. The tasks we had set ourselves – agreeing limits of care, completing a DNACPR form – were unfinished. 'Not today,' I said to the team. 'Not today.'

Sometimes the situation will not allow you to have the conversation properly, yet urgency pushes you into doing it anyway.

I remember giving a non-English speaking patient some bad news. She did not speak a word of English, and her own language was an unusual one. I had established that there were no relatives around; none of my medical or nursing colleagues spoke the relevant language, nor did any of the house-keeping staff; I would have to use LanguageLine.

Could I, should I, have postponed the conversation? This is a tricky point. She required a series of urgent investigations and procedures. She was caught in a whirlwind of activity. New clinical information had arisen in the last 12 hours. She had to be told what was going on. It was not realistic to postpone the conversation for three or four hours. Nor was it appropriate to call her closest friend and ask them to interpret over the phone – for they would be hearing the bad news and communicating it back to the patient simultaneously. So... the phone. It did not have speaker mode.

I introduced myself. Handed over the phone.

I asked what she knew. Handed over the phone.

I said that the scan on admission had shown some worrying changes in the pancreas. Handed over the phone.

She nodded, but I saw her expression alter from innocent curiosity to bewilderment, then deep concern.

I said that we were very worried about the possibility of cancer, but we weren't a hundred percent sure yet, hence the need for further tests today, and another procedure to help the symptoms. Handed over the phone.

Tears formed over her lower eyelids. She looked at me. The remove, the fact that my words had been processed by a third party, made it more difficult to find the correct emotional response. The nurse who was present placed a hand on the patient's arm, a gesture that needed no translation. The junior doctor tapped a version of the exchange into the electronic record.

I said it was too soon to talk about the sort of definitive treatment that might be required; we needed a biopsy and to review the next scan result. Handed over the phone.

I asked if she wanted to ask me anything. Handed over the phone. Clearly, her mind was teeming with questions, doubts and fears. But now was not the time. This exchange was about raw information, planning the next steps, preparing the ground... but so cold, so 'clinical'.

She asked a couple of questions. She handed over the phone.

We were done.

I walked away feeling that I – we – had done a bad job. A phenomenally bad job. There she was with no one to talk to, until a friend arrived who spoke the same, unusual language. Complete isolation.

There are times when you know that you have done harm. You walk away feeling like a wrecker.

I came to see a female patient who had been admitted several times over the last few months. It wasn't cancer, and as is often the case in 'benign' conditions, neither her GP nor the many other doctors who had met her in hospital had recognised the features of approaching death. After the usual business of the ward round I paused, took the temperature of the situation, made a silent assessment of the patient's ability to handle the discussion and sat on her bed. Her husband was sitting in a chair on the other side of the bed. I could tell by his expression and general demeanour that he knew what I was going to say even before I started.

Within minutes of making it clear to them that the repeated admissions were signs that her body was failing, a pall had settled across the cubicle. When I said that we needed to consider what would happen if her heart were to stop, there were tears. It was as though I had broken the news that she was dying – right now. Yet this was a preparatory conversation, an attempt to allow her to let us know her views weeks and months before that happened. It was an attempt to get the couple to face reality, an undeniable reality, before it rushed at them so quickly that the decisions were also rushed, confused or taken completely out of their hands. Yet it felt like I was single-handedly wrecking her life, pulling out the last vestiges of optimism and throwing them on the floor.

Another relative came onto the ward; her husband heard the voice outside and called, 'No, don't come in, wait outside,' as though the conversation we were having was a turning point. The *big* conversation. Yet the point of such conversations is that they do not take place at the point of inflexion, but before... way before the final emergency.

We finished. I completed the ward round. 45 minutes later, I passed the hospital cafeteria and saw the husband and the other, female relative sitting gloomily at a table, their faces red and tearstained. The impact of the conversation had been huge. It had made visible the monster that had been growing for two years. It had made inescapable the decisions that had to be confronted sooner rather than later. It had caused acute emotional distress and accelerated the grieving process. As I walked past the cafeteria, the husband noticed me and stared blankly. I acknowledged him, but there was no right way to act, and I moved on.

It had been *my* decision to start talking. It would have been so much easier to ignore it, to discharge the patient after she recovered from the present emergency, and let nature take its course. Then, when she was deteriorating in a way that any person, medical or not, could see was a prelude to death, another doctor would have to confront the issue. So much easier.

Yet, a few days later, when the emotional injury settled, I met her husband again by the entrance to the ward. He thanked me for being 'honest'. That is the doctor's reward for choosing to start the conversation. It is meagre. But attached to it is the knowledge that when a patient does enter the terminal phase, the necessary decisions will have been taken, or at least considered. The patient's wishes will have been explored while they still had the capacity to think clearly and the ability to articulate them. The doctor who started the conversation probably won't be there to witness the benefits of that hard conversation. Although they walked away feeling as though they had wrecked a life, they may well have done the opposite, encouraging the patient to rebuild and construct a new approach, a different way of thinking, better suited to the challenges that come in the last weeks and months of life.

Choosing the right words in the gravest of circumstances is perhaps the ultimate challenge.

2.6 Loose

Great examination. Amanda's liver was grossly enlarged, its bumpy edge palpable just under the skin of her abdomen. But she looked well and wasn't even aware of the anatomical extremity that she had been growing since the day she was born. Her liver was packed full of cysts. They were benign and represented no real danger.

When I asked her specific questions, there were some clues. About a year ago, she had begun to feel full halfway through her meals. She has lost some weight as a result and it was this complaint that had led her to the GP, who had then very sensibly arranged an ultrasound scan.

'You have quite a rare condition. Polycystic liver disease. It affects about 1 in 100,000 people. Sometimes the kidneys are affected too, but not in your case.'

She asked about the risk of cancer, of rupture, of bleeding. All good questions. I was reassuring and suggested that she come back in six months. If the liver was pressing in on the stomach and causing her to lose more weight, she might need something surgical. But that was unlikely.

'Oh, and there's something else. There is an association with aneurysms in the brain... these are blood vessels that have weak walls and develop into swellings. If they rupture it can be very dangerous, so I will arrange a brain scan for you.'

Her face whitened. She was scared.

'It's very rare,' I said, trying to reassure.

Arranging the scan was difficult. Our radiology department scrutinised each request very carefully, and if the reason for doing it was insufficient (in the opinion of the senior radiologist), a request could be cancelled. In fact the radiologist rang me two weeks later.

'We don't recommend these scans unless there are symptoms you know...'

I tried to talk her into it, but she would not move. I rang a neurologist for back up. Five weeks had passed by now.

'I wouldn't do a scan unless there is a family history of cerebral haemorrhage or stroke,' he explained.

'But I told her I would get a scan...'

'Yes.' he replied, enigmatic but unhelpful.

Life and other patients displaced the issue from my mind. Three months after the first appointment, Amanda returned to my clinic. Her mouth was rigid with anger.

'I looked up aneurysms. They can kill you, or you can end up disabled. I've been thinking about it every day, every single day. I could barely work for a month. And I haven't had the scan...'

I apologised. I explained that I had discussed her case with a specialist, and that in his opinion, a scan was required only if someone in her family had suffered a brain haemorrhage.

'But what if I *do* have one? I won't know until it bursts, will I?'

There followed a grovelling, 10-minute apology. I shouldn't have mentioned the risk of aneurysms without checking the expert guidance. I recognised that I had, by loosely introducing the spectre of brain haemorrhage, ruined two or three months of her life. Incomplete knowledge had led to a psychologically damaging, open-ended situation. I was sorry. I really was. But I could not take back the anxiety that I had heaped onto her.

She calmed down. She never did get the brain scan. And I have never mentioned aneurysms in this context again, unless my vague inquiries into their family history ('Any strokes, heart attacks?') happened to elicit a positive response.

2.7 Signals

The average ward round in an ED or acute medical unit will require one or several 'proper' sit down conversations, ideally in a room or private space, so that the doctor can discuss all eventualities. Such discussions, in my experience, are reserved for situations in which the patient appears to be dying, clearly pre-terminal, or at significant risk of suffering a cardiac arrest from which he or she will not be successfully resuscitated by CPR. The conversation with relatives will explain that the short-term prognosis is poor, and that CPR may not be inappropriate. But uncertainty requires a different kind of conversation, one that takes place at a less profound emotional level and does not usually cause the clinician to invoke the full panoply of communication skills. As we saw in 'Cruel', uncertainty leads to a 'preparatory' conversation, and usually takes place at the bedside. The challenge is to balance clarity with mere suggestion, frankness with compassion and the risk of information overload with a comprehensive exploration of possible eventualities. Not only this; the messages conveyed must also be understood by all of those present – the patient (often elderly), a spouse and sometimes younger members of the family. They may interpret words and signals very differently.

An 86-year-old man has been admitted with pneumonia. His exercise tolerance is quite poor (a hundred yards, slowly), perhaps due to chronically diseased lungs. He had a major heart attack 10 years ago but got over it. The chest x-ray shows a large area of infection, but he is talking and jovial. He has received antibiotics and requires a modest amount of oxygen.

The conversation, with the patient, his wife and a daughter, may go like this:

Doctor: It looks like a chest infection.

Patient: OK, doctor. Is that all?

Doctor: Pneumonia...

Patient (recognising this word as a graver condition): Oh!

Doctor: That's we call chest infections. It's a serious illness. Because your lungs are already a bit scarred it could go on to make you quite ill.

Wife: So it's serious then?

Doctor: It is, pneumonia is always serious. But it should respond to the antibiotics.

Patient: That's alright then...

Daughter: What do you mean by 'serious', doctor?

Doctor: It could get worse, if the infection spreads.

Daughter: And then what will you do?

Doctor: If his breathing deteriorates, and his oxygen levels fall...that would be a very worrying development.

Daughter: What would happen?

Doctor: Well...sometimes patients need more help with their breathing...

Daughter: A ventilator you mean?

Doctor: Perhaps, but we would need to ask the intensive care doctors to come and see your dad and tell us what sort of treatments would help...

Wife: He doesn't seem that unwell now, doctor.

Doctor: No, he's tolerating the infection very well. It's just I think it's important that you know that pneumonia is a potentially serious illness, and patients can get worse before they get better...

Daughter: He barely sees his doctor you know. There's nothing really wrong with him.

Doctor: That is very encouraging, but the x-ray does show some signs of damage from before the infection, and that's why I'm being a bit cautious...

There are oblique phrases in here, some of which are not entirely honest if we examine the thoughts behind them:

> *'quite ill'* – the doctor means *'critically ill'*
> *'worrying development',* meaning *'life threatening deterioration'*
> *'patients can get worse before they get better...',* meaning, in fact, *'not all who get worse will get better'*
> *'It's just I think it's important that you know',* meaning *'I really want you to take this in; I'm really worried'*
> *'tell us what sort of treatments would help',* meaning *'I can't commit to escalation to intensive care and mechanical ventilation; it's not entirely my decision...but nor do I want to engage on an escalation of care discussion at this moment...'*
> *'cautious',* meaning *'I'm very worried about your father; there's a real possibility that this infection will prove fatal.'*

Why use these oblique terms? Why not be clear, and say what he is thinking? Because the doctor has to be cautious in both directions – not too encouraging or unrealistically positive, but not too gloomy or doom-laden either. For after all, the doctor has only just met the patient and the family, and as I explained above, there is not yet enough evidence to justify an end-of-life type discussion.

Should the doctor discuss resuscitation? Yes, probably, but his reticence on this issue will be equally understandable. The patient is independent usually, limited yes, but with a good quality of life. And as his daughter says, there is little in the way of formally established or active co-morbidities. He may well have chronic airways disease, but no one has told him so. There is not enough in the history to convince the consultant that he should be 'Not For Resuscitation'.

The result of all these deliberations? – neither one thing nor the other. Subtle hints, tangential phrases that may be interpreted by the daughter in one way and the patient or his wife in another. The patient may be transferred to the medical ward reassured that the antibiotics will make him better, the daughter may go home worrying about the consultant's thinly veiled pessimism, or 'caution'. And the doctor walks on to the next patient thinking he has sent out enough cautionary signals to cover all the bases. How wrong they might be.

2.8 Privacy

Ward patients sometimes comment on, or complain about, the fact that they can hear conversations between doctors and other patients through the curtains. When you're having a conversation with a patient, you may as well imagine that the room is entirely open plan; curtains provide a visual barrier, but are more of a symbol of privacy, like the sheets hung in overcrowded homes of centuries past. Imagining the bay as a small hall with six or eight beds arranged in it makes you think twice about having any conversations at all, yet to conduct every sensitive conversation in a private room would be impractical. This begs the question: what kind of conversations are acceptable on the ward, and which should be reserved for a truly private space?

We are used to making special arrangements for breaking very bad news, end-of-life or DNACPR conversations, and for planned conferences where several family members are expected. To gather four or five plastic chairs around a bed in a cramped space and pretend to be comfortable delving into intimate and existentialist details is inappropriate. But other conversations, the majority, are conducted within earshot of strangers. Sometimes, a 'routine' conversation about treatment (which is still, after all, highly personal), can transform into something else.

In conversation with a jaundiced, alcohol-dependent patient called Mr Jeffries, I sensed a complete lack of understanding about the seriousness of his situation. I was standing next to his bed. Other members of the firm, a nurse, and a student, stood nearby, listening or typing into computers on wheels. We had been talking about the next set of tests, progress, plans. Nothing too personal, nothing too sensitive. Then I took the conversation into a darker place, to emphasise the gravity of his illness.

'I'll be truthful with you, Mr Jeffries. And it's a lot easier for me to say than for you to do, I know, but if you start drinking again after you get home, you will probably die in the next three months.' It took him unawares. His eyes moistened with the realisation of how close to death he was. The visit ended, and the nurse stayed with him to provide comfort and make our disappearance from the bedside less abrupt.

As I drew the curtain back, I looked across to the patient opposite, who had of course heard everything. Now he knew as much about the alcoholic patient's poor prognosis as the patient himself. As patient 2 looked across at patient 1, there was shared, highly personal knowledge. Patient 1 was left totally exposed. It felt wrong. It was wrong. Yet, how could I have done this better? Perhaps I should have paused the *conversation* and said, 'We really need to talk about the future, in private... how about I come back later...' But there was no 'later' that day. I could have delegated the task to a very capable registrar, but that also felt wrong. And the conversation just went in that direction, naturally.

Hospital is a harsh leveller. It is difficult for the great machine to tailor and modulate its processes to the individual sensitivities of each patient. What one patient would regard as unacceptable in terms of privacy, another will have no problems with. As doctors and nurses, we tend to apply our own standard to everyone. Yet that standard has probably been lowered by brutal shifts in ED where people display their vulnerability to all and sundry in waiting rooms and scream in pain or cry inches from strangers. It is easy, as a doctor, to think 'the priority here is treatment; this is a busy environment, and dignity comes second...'

Nurses are the guardians of dignity. Yet doctors can with an irritated scowl or a quick glance at their watch, overrule the gentle suggestion that 'it might be better to have this conversation away from the bedside...' I know I have done that. A conversation that I think is 'ward-appropriate' might, in a nursing colleague's mind, touch on a subject that no other patient should be allowed to hear. Who decides? Does the acuity of the ward, or the incessant flow of humanity through an Acute Medical Unit, justify a reduction in privacy thresholds?

There is no list of topics that should be explored in true privacy. The patient should, in theory, be in control. To discover a patient's level of sensitivity, it is necessary to ask at the beginning, 'I'd like to talk about x, y and z; would you rather we did this somewhere else?' The danger, perhaps, is that they will say yes! Then it will be necessary to move everyone.

As ever, the solution starts with a patient-centred view, and empathy. What would you feel if you were told you have three months to live in a room where five other patients could, if they were alert enough and unable to switch off their ears, hear every word? Like all things in medicine, quality takes more time, more patience... it requires the machine to slow down.

2.9 Unwanted

Helen lay on a trolley in the ED. So far, the care had been good. Her leg still hurt, but the staff seemed to be getting on with things – taking blood, injecting antibiotics, dressing the horrible wound through which bacteria had gained access to her system. When would they put her in proper bed, though? They hadn't yet decided which ward to send her to; that seemed to be the problem. The trolley was hard and narrow. Her arms were pressed against the cold metal of the side-rails. And the noise! So many people calling out or giving instructions.

A voice she recognised pierced the hubbub. A man's voice, distinctive. It was the doctor who had come down to examine her leg. Her doctor! She could just about make out his shape through the gap in the curtain. He was on the phone, and he was agitated. She followed his words. Of course, Helen could only hear half the conversation.

'No. Sorry, but no. It's not surgical, there's no way this lady will need surgical management...'

A pause.

'It doesn't matter what the protocol says, I'm not accepting her. There's no compartment syndrome, no bony involvement...'

Another pause.

'Well, call my consultant if you like, I'm not taking her onto my list. There's no indication. She'll just sit on our ward getting antibiotics; my consultant won't want to see her; she's got other complex problems that need medical care... no!'

He hung up. A more junior colleague, a female doctor, joined him. He gestured emphatically in Helen's direction and said,

'In future please don't accept referrals like that. I've had to turf[11] her back to medics, they started going on about what if she needs plastic surgery or debridement. We can come and give an opinion if her foot goes bad, but we're not having her on our list. Waste of time.'

He walked away from the station and passed Helen's bay. He kept his eyes down, but Helen followed him with her gaze and made the briefest of eye contact when he glanced in. The doctor smiled weakly. He had no idea that she had heard him. He carried on walking, but Helen called out,

'Ah, doctor!' He stopped and stood by the curtain.

'Yes, Mrs. Thomas?'

'So will you be looking after me? Am I going to your ward?'

'Errr... no. The kind of infection you have is best looked after by the medical team. I'm a surgeon, so I've asked that the medical team look after you on their ward.'

'I see. But they said I might need an operation on the wound. It's very severe.'

'We can always do that later if need be. But you're better off under the medical doctors to start with.' He moved on, but before he was out of earshot Helen muttered,

'I wouldn't want to be a waste of time.'

The doctor slowed for an instant, then carried on. Helen had no idea whether he felt bad, embarrassed, or if he just didn't care.

We all know that negotiation over the ownership of patients is a reality. Imagine if they could hear the arguments that sometimes take place. That is what I have done here – imagine a sad scenario in which a patient hears 'her doctor' doing his best to wash his hands of her. I'm not sure if such accidental indiscretions have occurred in reality; I suspect they have because such conversations occur many times, every day.

Medical diagnosis and early management are not clear-cut exercises and working out which teams should look after patients can take time. Robust conversations take place in which doctors explain why they should, or more commonly should not, take responsibility. If it's a 50:50 call, it can come down to pure assertiveness. Or, sometimes, the heartfelt intervention by a senior nurse who recognises that 'someone's got to look after this poor lady! Sort yourselves out!'

It may be shocking for non-medical readers to hear that patients are not automatically welcomed onto the lists of medical teams. It sounds inhumane. Yet there can be good reasons. The worst thing for a patient is to be admitted under a team that is inexpert in the management of their medical condition. This can lead to delays, avoidable deterioration or even clinical disengagement. It is important to be taken over by the most appropriate team, but determining which team this is can be a struggle.

There are unseemly struggles behind the scenes in many customer-, client- or user-facing organisations. In acute and emergency medicine, where patients are experiencing vulnerability and disempowerment, any sense of rejection is bound to have a very negative effect. So, doctors, next time you feel the need to argue over a referral and start horse-trading over individuals, imagine what impact your words might have on the patient, should they accidentally hear you!

2.10 Low

It's 9.15 AM. The medical team is full of energy and caffeine. We have patients to see, some of whom are on the road to recovery, others who have already been recognised as dying, and some who have uncertain futures. There are three new patients whose condition could worsen at any time. Given their frailty, I believe CPR would be futile. It is now my job to start a discussion about their future care. Three conversations. I take a deep breath.

The trainee doctors are attentive and still learning how to do this. I complete my assessment for the first patient, pause, then open the discussion. My version is not perfect, and it varies. If it does not vary, then it shows I am just repeating some learned lines – an impression that is important to avoid.

I open the patient's mind to the possibility of dying (be it suddenly or gradually). Their next of kin may be present. Each patient reacts in their own way. A faraway look is not uncommon. Sometimes a film develops over the eyes, glistening in the light of the nearby window. Poetry has no place here, but as a human, I am affected by the impact of my words.

This patient and I reach an understanding – we agree – that CPR is not the right thing to do if their heart stops. If either they or a relative had disagreed, we would park it, and arrange to speak about it again later. Now I walk away, unsure how to close the interaction. A hand on the arm, a swish of the curtain? There is no comfortable way, to be honest.

Outside the bay, we complete the DNACPR form to make it official, for the benefit of others who might be called to see the patient in an emergency.

For the next patient, we review her history and agree we need to anticipate the worst, even if – fingers crossed – it doesn't happen during this admission.

I use subtly different words but move in the same direction. This time there is a more overt reaction, and a longer discussion. The thought of dying has never crossed her mind. Nor her husband's. I recall the young man with spinal muscular atrophy, described earlier in 'Paralysis'. The damage that can be done if people shy away from hard conversations. Part of me brims with anger: she has an incurable, gradually worsening condition, and has been seen by her GP and in specialist clinics umpteen times over the past year. Why has no one brought this up? Why does it have to be me? I could just leave it. She might not deteriorate after all. Why not leave it until she does?

But if that happens at 3am, and a foundation year doctor is asked to see her, and they refer to a registrar who has never met the patient, there will be hurried decision-making; the patient will probably not be conscious enough to express their wishes; an ICU consultant will be asked to make a call based on scant information. It's bad medicine, just like the cases reviewed by National confidential Enquiry into Patient outcome and Death (NCEPOD): of 198 patients who in the opinion of an expert panel, should have had a DNACPR decision, only 22 did (11%). For the remaining patients, CPR was predictably futile.

The conversation must happen now. Encouraging doctors to start these conversations, and training them how to do it, is vital. Even more important is raising awareness among patients who may be approaching the last year of life, so they can start the conversation with loved ones.

This conversation has taken half an hour. Not long in the life of the patient, relative to the magnitude of the subject under discussion. But very long in the context of a ward round. Never mind. The time must be taken.

We come to the third patient.

I enter the bed space. The visit proceeds along routine lines while I make a general assessment. Then I reach a fork in the path. Now is the time to level with them. But I am not up to it. I have left two patients in mute distress (how could it be otherwise?). I have reformulated the words to keep them fresh and sincere and specific to them. I have struck a balance between brutal realism (I'm not one for drawing a vivid picture of CPR, but the act has to be mentioned) and sensitivity. I have asked myself, as we continued our progress along the ward, if I am being too pessimistic. If the other doctors they saw didn't bring up dying, perhaps I shouldn't either? I make a decision. Not today. Another day. Let's talk about it on Wednesday. I haven't got the energy. The emotional tank is empty. Or I'll ask the registrar to do it, she's good.

'So is he still for resus?' asks the nurse, who needs clarity. It is she who will have to call the crash team if there is a collapse.

'Yes.'

'Even if he deteriorates? He looks so … frail.'

'We'll cross that bridge when we come to it. Sorry.'

And so we move on, hoping that the worst doesn't happen before we find the time and the energy – a very specific form of energy – to broach the subject.

2.11 Edge

There isn't time to go into every 'complaint' (symptom) in a typical clinic. There just isn't. So, however open my initial question ('How are things?'), I narrow down to the important matter quickly. Most patients understand this, and tacitly agree to drop other concerns. It sounds like bad medicine; it is certainly non-holistic, but it is real life. If symptoms unconnected to the condition that brings a patient to the clinic are explored for too long, less time will be spent pursuing the potentially dangerous diagnosis. Therefore, patients receive little more than sympathy and a recommendation that they had 'better see your GP about that.'

Sometimes patients insist, though. When this happens, it is necessary to find the language that combines genuine interest (after all, to dismiss something that causes anxiety is just rude) and skilful management of the time-limited interaction. However, if despite the nuanced nods, silences and redirections, the primary issue continues to be relegated to the background, less subtle tactics are required. Perhaps,

'Sorry, Mr _____, we really should concentrate on what your GP wrote to me about,' Or, 'I can tell that's causing you some real problems, but I'll have to ask your GP to refer you to another clinic...'

I had finished examining the patient and was sitting at the desk, looking at x-rays and blood results, trying to work out what tests to arrange next. From the couch my patient returned for the third time to an irrelevant (to my mind, trivial) complaint. Filtering his words ruthlessly while I concentrated on the most efficient path to a final diagnosis, I mumbled something half-hearted and non-committal. There was a pause. He rose from the couch and said,

'Oh, *forget* about it then.'

The sharp edge to his words pulled me out from the clinical, impersonal space into which I had fallen. One rarely hears such a tone. I saw that I had been rude. I turned in the swivel chair and back-pedalled desperately,

'No, it's important! Sorry! Have a seat. We need to think about how you can get it sorted...'

Gradually, the consultation was retrieved. Left as it was, the encounter would have gone the way of many hospital appointments – into the 'he/she barely listened to me' category. We discussed the other matter, and I promised to do something. He left content (I think; I hope). The appointment overran. But I owed him that, for losing sight of what mattered to him, and steering too close to the edge of a precipice down which trust can easily be lost.

2.12 Dance

On every ward round he looks up (though I try to meet his gaze from an equal height, sitting on the bed) and finds the positives. He presumes there is a surgical cure, though I know already that it cannot be. He welcomes the idea of chemotherapy – it worked so well last time – but I know it can offer nothing more than a brief extension.

He is 48. He lives on hope as the fatally undermined airplane flies on fumes, its passengers observing the steady passage of the clouds in deep, sweet ignorance. I believe that the face he wears to meet the face of his wife, that 'we can deal with this' mask, can be fixed by no other kind of glue. He thinks she needs to hear that there is a future, so his mind cannot admit of any alternative. That is my amateur psychological analysis. But I have seen her leaving the cubicle, how the thin smile straightens as she turns away into the outside world, and I think that she knows. She does not know the facts, but she recognises death in her husband's sunken features.

I am too negative. The modern way is never to say there is no hope, that 'nothing can be done'. There are many things we can do; there is much that we can offer. Palliative care is a specialty, a branch of medicine as established now as cardiology or oncology. We will treat you. Yes, yes, yes, of course you will. But you can't save me, can you? They see through our pretense. Come on! When you're 48 and dying of cancer, you don't want to hear how great the palliative care is. Do you?

I don't know. I'm not dying.

The problem with this chap is that he's been through it before. This is a recurrence. In another hospital, at a preposterously young age, he got pancreatic cancer. Another hospital, another country, another hemisphere, in fact. They did a good job, technically. Cut out the tumour, replaced a major abdominal vein with a graft, replumbed an adjacent artery. When I read the op notes (lifted from his impeccably kept folder), I sighed. It must have been edging into those vessels. Locally advanced, as we say. And far too many nodes. Of the seven they removed, six contained cancer. But they hammered him with chemo, cleaned the circuits of any rogue cells, got him through a few bouts of neutropenia, and gave him the all-clear. Cured.

He was never cured.

It was bound to return. Ask any pancreatic surgeon, they will shake their head. Locally advanced, nodal spread. Borrowed time.

He was not aware. He had been feeling odd for two or three months now, and it did not occur to him that it might have come back. Even now, in this hospital, he seems not to know that so manifest a recurrence of symptoms (he is jaundiced; the cancer is blocking off his liver) can mean only one thing.

I want to ring that highly skilled surgeon on the other side of the world and ask him (I read the op notes; it's a he) – 'What were you playing at, letting him think he was cured? Didn't you know what the prognosis was? You let him go back to his family, move jobs, live his life, with no idea that what is happening now was inevitable. All the plans he made, all the images he entertained. False. All false. Built on a foundation of lies. No, not lies, that's too strong. Just the absence of truth. You let the best-case scenario flower into a confirmed reality. And now it's crashing down around him.'

If I ever see him – in some sunny pancreatic conference, on some doctor-packed airplane – I will tell him this directly. Look at the mess you left for me to clear up. Me. For it is I who must now sit with him, tomorrow, perhaps next week, when all the facts are in place and all the opinions have been given, to dismantle the delicate construction that occupies his deluded mind. That reaching tower around which winged visions flutter and speak of future milestones, his daughter's next birthday party, the work that needs to be done on the house, that second home. Future life. A life which I, the messenger, must now take away.

The messenger. Brings to mind a line from *Anthony and Cleopatra*. I saw it with my wife around the time this patient was on my ward. Ralph Fiennes was the lead. A messenger, quaking, comes to tell the Egyptian queen that her love has betrayed her in taking a wife. 'I that do bring the news made not the match,' he says, to Cleopatra's threat that the bearer of bad news 'shalt be whipp'd with wire, and stew'd in brine, smarting in lingering pickle.' A good night it was. My wife's hand lay in mine, both of us enjoying a rare excursion. A good life, a London life, privileged. Why do I tell you this? Because as I sat there, before the spectacle, he, the poor He of this piece, floated across my field of vision from stage left. Lying in bed, yellow with jaundice, his face tense with pain, smarting from the puncture that my colleagues in radiology had made in his side to drain the bile ducts. That's how I left him on Friday night, before throwing on my scarf and heading off to the theatre. I left him waiting for morphine.

I know the How. There will be a specialist nurse, hopefully an oncologist too. I will compress his future between my honest hands using carefully chosen words laced in maximum empathy. We will advise that he has four to six months with chemo or two, maybe less, without. (I wouldn't take that deal, personally.) We will remain positive, talking of all that can be done. He will see through it. Then I will watch the mask begin to crumble, like a petrified monster tapped by the hero's sword, falling away to form a pile of grey powder on the floor.

What about the When? Tomorrow. I have danced around it for too long. There are no more behind-the-scene negotiations to be had. The multi-disciplinary team meeting has reached its consensus – no surgery, no cure. Every hour that passes without honest communication adds to the deceit. We know what he does not. Have known, for days. Since before the play, to be honest. There have been whispered conversations outside the bay. Yesterday the nurse in charge of the ward asked me, 'Have you discussed resus status?' No. NO! That comes later, after I have confirmed to him that there is no cure. Be patient. But it is a sign. He looks bad now, his energy is failing. The nurses' senses are attuned to the possibility of crisis. It has gone on for too long, this black tango. It cannot be allowed to continue.

He knew.

I told them nothing – he and his wife – that they did not know.

It was I who was walking in the dark.

You know something? My amateur psychological analysis leads me to conclude that he was protecting me, the messenger. He saw me dancing with words, he read my evasions, and he waited for me. Waited until I was ready. And he was kind to the messenger. Too kind.

3

Skin: Resilience

Judging by what you have read so far, you would be forgiven for thinking that this medical career has been a litany of grief, some of it my patients' and some mine. Yet I carried on and seemed genuinely to enjoy the work. Dare I say it, I actually thrived. How can this be?

Not all doctors thrive in the face of bad outcomes. Some decide they must leave the profession. Adam Kay, in his best-selling book *'This Is Going to Hurt'*,[12] describes how he gave up medicine after his involvement in a caesarean section that went very wrong. He was clearly dissatisfied from the beginning, and this incident was the final straw. Most doctors find a way to get over the setbacks. Some associate this with 'resilience', the property of things to absorb pressure and retain their natural shape. Others hate this word (of which more later), because it puts the responsibility to succeed or fail squarely on the shoulders of the doctor, not the system in which they work. In this part of the book, I will describe some of the ways in which I reacted to bad events and explore how those reactions helped me carry on.

3.1 Right

Being an effective doctor requires a mixture of assertiveness and sensitivity to others' opinions. As we saw in Part II, you must be receptive to the ideas of those around you, but if you think you are right, if you *know* you are right and you believe the patient will suffer if your plan is not followed, then you must have the courage of your convictions.

Mrs. Mary Obade, 78 years old, came to the hospital with abdominal pain. There were signs of infection in the blood tests, and her arterial blood was mildly acidic (due to lactic acid, a substance we will hear more of later in the sad case of Jake Adcock). Her kidneys failed, and she was transferred to ICU for haemofiltration. Her liver wasn't great either, so I was asked to see her. She was in pain and could barely concentrate on my questions. When I pressed her abdomen she winced. The ICU consultant arrived at the bedside through the drawn curtains and asked me my opinion.

'Looks like mesenteric ischaemia to me.' In this condition, the blood supply to the bowel is blocked by clots or cholesterol-laden plaques. The only treatment, once it has progressed to 'dead gut', is major surgery to remove the affected length of bowel before it begins to go gangrenous. In advanced cases, the bowel looks grey or black when it is lifted out of the abdominal incision; sometimes, it just falls apart in the surgeon's hand.

'No. The CT ruled it out.' replied the consultant.

DOI: 10.1201/9781003189824-3

'I know, but that was done 36 hours ago. I'd suggest another one today.'

He winced, in clear disagreement. 'You don't think it's cholangitis?' This is an infection in the bile ducts.

'Not really, too much pain, not enough jaundice. Have the surgeons seen her?'

'Yes. They don't think there's an indication to operate.'

'What about a laparoscopy, just to look inside and see if there's any dead gut?'

'They didn't think there was a surgical issue.'

The end.

What should I do? My instinct was: this lady has bowel ischaemia and is at risk of becoming even more unwell. We disagreed. Should I make a fuss, jump up and down? How sure was I, really?

'Well, my suggestion is you get another CT scan today, see if anything has changed.' And I left. You asked for my opinion, there it is. Do what you want. You're looking after her; she's not my responsibility.

Next morning I saw her again. Even more tender, but the blood tests had improved, and the blood was less acidic. But no new CT scan.

'Are you going to scan her?' I asked the consultant.

'If her condition changes.'

'She's very tender. There's something not right in there.'

'We'll monitor.'

'Well, you know what I think. Clinically, she is worse, even though the blood tests are a bit better. I strongly advise re-imaging.'

Next day I could not see her until the afternoon. When I arrived on the ICU, there were more machines and infusions around her. The ICU consultant walked over.

'Ah, good afternoon, Dr Right!'

'What happened?'

'She deteriorated last night, her abdomen began to distend, the on-call surgeon came to see her and took her straight to theatre. She took out 90 cm of dead small bowel.'

'Wow.'

'So, you were right.'

'Well, it's a hard diagnosis. She got surgery when she needed it.'

'Mmmmm.'

It felt good, of course, to be vindicated. But I wondered, as I looked at the charts and saw that she had come close to cardiac arrest on the night of her deterioration, if I should have sought out the surgeon 24 hours earlier and pushed hard for an operation. The patient would probably have lost far less bowel, and her recovery would have been faster. As it was, there was no guarantee that she would survive this: she was in four-organ failure and her age was against her.

Why didn't I push harder?

Quite simply, I didn't fancy the battle. I didn't want to go head-to-head. I didn't want to make too much trouble. To make a strong case for surgery, as a non-surgeon myself, would have cost me emotionally, and perhaps reputationally. On the other hand, if I had pushed hard and been rebuffed, my reputation would be even stronger now, having been proved right.

Reputation. Was this all I was concerned about? No, not only that. I had concluded that now was not the time to go full-guns. The condition was outside my direct area of expertise; I needed to be standing on firmer ground before entering battle. That time would come, I was sure of it. Mary Obade had the benefit of several experienced doctors, and my opinion was just one of those. There was no need for me to feel bad. Ultimately, though it pains me to admit it, I needed to look after my own skin.

3.2 Wall

Valerie, 79 years old, was admitted with bleeding oesophageal varices (complicating a previously undiagnosed liver disorder). Varices are swollen veins, as thick as your little finger, that run up the inside of the oesophagus. Their walls become thin over time, and often they rupture. The blood pours out, filling the stomach. Patients vomit pure, dark blood; it is one of the most frightening experiences imaginable. They can die within hours. That's what happened to Sarah, in 'Comfort'.

I performed an endoscopy. It took 45 minutes and was hard work, but I convinced myself that I had sealed the culprit blood vessel with an elastic band. It was early in my specialist training and I was still proving myself, but I made the decision not to back myself up by calling for help or inserting an inflated balloon to ensure that the vessels remained compressed overnight. Next day I came back to work... and she was gone. My gut seized. The first question I asked in handover was, 'Did she bleed?' The answer was 'No – it was a heart attack... could have happened at any time'. Relief, endorphins, dopamine, whatever, flooded over me. Relief before grief. I realised that a doctor's first reaction, on hearing about an unexpected death, is to ask themselves – *did I do anything wrong?* I feared blame.

The same sensation occurred with Mr Braithwaite, the man with oesophageal cancer who I described in 'Listen'. Having learned about his diagnosis, I went back to the notes and re-read every letter that I had written. I scrutinised them looking for justification. Was each decision logical, given the available information? Was I vulnerable? Would I be able to explain the rationale behind my decision not to arrange another endoscopy if cross-examined by a coroner?

I was building a wall – a wall of justification.

I had seen it before, in other people, in even more dramatic situations. As a student, I assisted a surgical registrar during an open cholecystectomy (removal of the gallbladder). I was holding back the liver with a steel retractor, and could see nothing of the operating field, partly because the incision was so modest. Instead, I watched the registrar's increasingly sweaty face. He muttered through the operation and cursed his inability to see the anatomical structures properly. Mid-sentence, he stopped talking. He took his hands out of the wound, clasped them over his gowned chest and walked over to the light box in the corner to study the images that were pinned there.

'I've cut the bile duct,' he said, with great simplicity. My slow brain tried to work out if this was a good or bad thing. He ripped off his gloves and picked up the black telephone in the corner of the room. He was calling his consultant. By this time, I had realised that cutting the bile duct is a very bad thing, for this leaves no channel through which the patient's liver can secrete bile. He should have cut the *cystic* duct. While his consultant attached the patient's jejunum to his biliary apparatus, through a far bigger incision, muttering things like 'Why, *why* did you cut it?' and 'How could you hope to see through that blasted small hole?'; the registrar, usually so bullish, was in quiet torment.

Next day I attended the usual early morning ward round. I expected to find him sheepish and withdrawn, but he was just the same. Confident, challenging, a good eye for detail, occasionally aggressive if the standards of the junior team appeared to have slipped. I was amazed. The pain of failure had washed over him. Later, in the coffee room, I overheard him talking to another consultant. He was explaining why the mistake had been made. The images on the x-ray were misleading; he had anticipated problems. He had consented the patient for conversion to an open operation, and a higher-than-average risk of complications. The gall bladder was diseased, stuck down, 'like glue, like concrete'; the other consultant nodded in understanding.

I understood. The surgical registrar, battered, standing at the edge of a cliff of self-doubt, had found a way to manage this challenge.

He had built a wall of *reasons*, and it was very strong.

3.3 Stick

As soon as I felt the deep sting of the needle as it entered my finger, I knew what it meant – potential disaster.

I was cutting a space between the ribs of a patient in intensive care, making room for the insertion of a large chest drain. The tissues were tough, and I had to tear at the fibres with my fingers deep under the skin. But the patient was not fully sedated, and she was feeling it despite the local anaesthetic injection I had administered beforehand.

Then, I did something stupid. I kept one finger in the cut, so as not to lose the track I had struggled to form, and with my other hand inserted the anaesthetic needle alongside the leading gloved index finger. In this way, I hoped to numb the deeper tissues. Instead, I jabbed my own fingertip – *ouch* ... a shock.

It was not the pain. It was the immediate fear that the hepatitis C virus in the patient's blood could now be running up the veins of my arm and into my bloodstream. I withdrew my finger, looked down at my hand, tore off the glove and squeezed the fingertip until droplets of blood came out.

The nurse helping me recognised what had happened but had nothing to say. I walked over to a sink, washed the blood off, wrapped a waterproof dressing around the tiny wound and went back to the patient. She still needed a chest drain after all.

Soon the job was done, and the rest of the nightshift passed without incident. But throughout the small hours, I could think only of myself: were there any viruses in the needle? How many would it take to cause a permanent infection? Would I need anti-viral treatment? Would it work? If it failed, would I develop cirrhosis; would I end up in this very hospital, waiting for a transplant?

I was distracted by anxiety for weeks, not to a disabling degree, not so as anyone would notice. But it gnawed at me.

Six weeks later, I had a blood test to see if there were detectable levels of virus in me. A week after that, I attended the occupational health department to get the result. The nurse had evidently not read a hepatitis C result before. She looked quizzically at the small piece of paper in front of her and tilted her head slightly.

'Err ... you have... err ... hepatitis C.'

I leaned over the desk and looked at the report closely, upside down. I turned the report round and saw that she had misread a < for a >. I had < 50 virus particles per millilitre of blood, not > 50. I was negative!

She accepted my interpretation and was embarrassed. I left the room and walked back to my ward. I felt 10 years older. My skin was cold and wet.

There were antibody tests at three and six months, and they were negative too. I was not infected. In fact, looking back, and knowing more about the statistics and the cleaning action that plastic gloves perform as a needle passes through them, it was never very likely. But the experience changed me.

Healthcare workers who have received needle stick injuries (NSI) can experience severe anxiety. In a study of 17 people who reacted so badly, they were referred to a psychiatric clinic; an acute stress reaction lasting up to two days was described, including acute anxiety, disbelief, physical tremor and inability to sleep. Three-quarters were diagnosed with an adjustment disorder, and a quarter met the criteria for post-traumatic stress disorder. Although my reaction was not so severe, I can certainly recognise some of the features in my own experience.

My NSI brought it home to me that while my career will involve me seeing hundreds or thousands of patients who might carry serious infections, there is only one of me. From that point on, I resolved to do everything I could to protect myself, not to a paranoid degree, but by applying a greater sense of caution.

Instead of plunging into the next cardiac arrest situation without a care for the bodily fluids that were leaking on to the patient's chest or bed, I held back until my gloves were safely on. That's what you're supposed to do anyway – universal precautions should be taken – but in real life, in emergencies, people often don't.

Not me, not anymore.

Beyond the arena of infection, I was less inclined to make sacrifices that might affect my health or put me at risk of making mistakes; swapping into crazy sequences of night and day shifts as a favour for colleagues, covering extra clinics when dog-tired, adding procedures to already busy lists – sensible behaviour, but a change.

The memory of that needle stick injury made me more cautious, a quality not always seen in younger doctors. Hesitancy deriving from self-centeredness is not expected in those who have entered a caring profession. But the fact is, medicine can put you in harm's way, and to stay well over a whole career means you must think twice before rushing in to help.

3.4 Distance

This will be a long one. There are several stories.

I watched an elderly male patient die. As ever, witnessing the transition between life and death caused me to pause. I did not know him well; I did not know his people. He was surrounded by the full crash team, which nowadays is a large group. As the attempt was abandoned and another consultant 'called it', I withdrew into the background. There was nothing I could do to help. I walked away to prepare my departure for a week-long break and couldn't help but think about him. His death. I wondered how it would affect me as I arrived home. The family were looking forward to seeing me, my return would mark the beginning of the 'real' holiday. I wanted to enter the house with a light spirit and smile. Yet, the image barely fading on my retina, and still vivid in my visual memory, was of a dead man.

How to separate the intensity of that memory from life outside the hospital? Detachment. That is the word, the process. An ability to cut the lines of emotion that stretch from the wards through the sliding doors, along the train track, the A-Road or cycle lane, thin but tenacious like the silk spun by Shelob, the giant spider-demon of Middle Earth. Pull as hard as you like, they don't snap. Yet, to avoid darkening our homes, they do need to be cut.

It is called detachment.

In 2013, a transplant surgeon called Simon Bramhall inscribed his initials on a patient's new liver with an argon beam tool used for cutting tissue. He had just performed a transplant operation. Because the liver failed (probably nothing to do with Mr Bramhall's skill), another surgeon was called in to remove it and put in a newly retrieved one. On lifting the failed liver out of the patient's body, the second surgeon saw the 4 cm high marks, 'SB'. It sounds bizarre and disrespectful. I know nothing of the people involved or any details beyond what was in the papers, but perhaps it exposes some interesting psychology.

In the medical specialties that require practical skill, especially surgery, you work hard to become an expert. Over the years, the movements of the hands and fingers become practised and slick. Operations that appear impossible to the lay person or junior trainee become routine, yet each patient is different. Each procedure presents its own challenges, hiccups, sudden recalibrations and extempore solutions. At the end of a particularly difficult case, when the patient appears stable and safe, you might sigh with relief, but also experience a surge of pride on a job well done. Congratulations are hard to come by in medicine. The job well done should be the norm, after all. But looking down at the organ, structure or vessel that now pulses healthily as a result of your dexterity, you might be forgiven for thinking – 'I did that!'

To mark a job well done with your initials is appropriate in other walks of life – in art and sculpture, in literature, in architecture. The artist owns the piece. A part of them, their skill, their creativity, their experience, lives within its lines.

Can medical procedures be regarded as art? Yes, I would say. The long facial reconstruction, the painstakingly re-joined finger, the delicately implanted heart valve… in the fine skill and seamless results, it is easy to identify the hallmarks of the inspired artisan, the committed artist. Perhaps it is understandable that a surgeon who comes to see the results of their skill as art feels the urge to sign it. In doing so, they detach the task from the person.

For it is a living body that we are talking about here. What lies under the skin is sovereign to the patient. They will carry it around with them for the rest of their lives. They were born with it. It is wholly theirs. (In the case of a transplanted liver of course, it belonged to another. The act of altruism and donation makes it worthy of even greater respect.) Perhaps that is the line that may have been crossed here – the distinction between what a surgeon can claim to 'own', and what is and will forever be sacred to the patient.

The following scenes explore other, more common forms of detachment. In the first two, I deal with a doctor's tendency to deal with one medical complaint only, separating it out from the whole person in order to limit the cognitive and emotional load.

i. *Scene: out-patient clinic*

'Hello, Mrs. Taylor, it's been what... 4 months... we were keeping an eye on the liver function, weren't we...' [Note the early effort to restrict discussion to the organ in which I specialise, and to the problem for which she was referred in the first place.]

'Yes, doctor, but...'

'How are you, generally?' [An open question, offered at some risk, to balance the early gambit]

'Not well, actually. My legs, they're aching so much, I can hardly leave the house sometimes...' [I look at the problem list, see 'peripheral vascular disease,' a complication no doubt of her diabetes, which is linked to her liver. Everything is connected.]

'Really. I'm sorry to hear that. Yes, you've got narrowed arteries, haven't you...'

'It's awful... awful... and they're numb. '

'That might be the nerves; they get affected in diabetes too...'

'What can I do?' [The tone is one of desperation. She is not asking what can be done, technically, medically, to the arteries in her legs, but to her life, which is a constant struggle.]

'I... what do you mean? '

'Well, I barely see anyone, and my back, my back is killing...'

'Your back.' [My tone is flat. Another issue now. The first hint of impatience.]

'It gets worse and worse; the mornings are awful...'

'And you've been to your GP about this?' [The first deflection.]

'Yes, but they don't want to x-ray it...'

A pause. I look at the liver tests on the screen.

'We need to talk about your liver, it's actually been very good recently...' [Trying to lighten things up.]

'I don't really know, doctor. If you say so.' [She has given up. She opened a window briefly into her difficulties, but she has seen how little interest I have in the things that matter to her.]

'Mrs. Taylor, Jean. I know there's a lot more going on that just your liver, though it's important we keep an eye on it. We need to. I know it's silent, it doesn't give you pain, but it's important. The other problems you have, I can see in the notes that you've seen various doctors here, specialists, about them....'

'But no one seems to know what's going on.' [This is the crux. She seeks a synthesis, perhaps even a meaning behind her suffering. Or a longer perspective. Or something else.]

'I'm sorry, Jean. I suppose your GP is in the best position to understand everything....' [I feel pathetic saying this. I am illustrating for her the medical model of primary and secondary care. I deal with my bit, the vascular surgeon deals with her bit, the diabetologist with another, and her GP, receiving multiple letters that explore in great detail each organ system but which probably all miss the larger point, tries to pull it all together. I must detach myself from her every problem. It is too much. And that is unsatisfactory, hence Mrs. Taylor's quiet desperation.]

It is time to close. We have already gone over the allotted 10 minutes.

'I'm going to arrange a new scan, some new blood tests… I'm encouraged, Jean. I know it's not easy, but things do look stable from my point of view.' [My narrow point of view.]

She nods. She knows she will get nothing more.

'I'll write to your GP, make sure they know how difficult you're finding things with your legs, and everything.'

She leaves.

I sigh. Bad job.

ii. *Scene: out-patient clinic*

The patient had undergone multiple investigations and several procedures during three stays in hospital. Her GP had referred her for a review on account of weight loss and worsening debility in the hope that something could be done to improve her condition. Her anxious family described how she had gone downhill, despite all that had been done. I nodded, unsurprised. That's what illness, infection and hospitalisation do. Then her husband said,

'And during all this time, nobody has really treated her as a whole person.'

I paused. Rather than letting the comment slip by, I asked him what he meant by that. Because everything that happened seemed logical and correct to me. Her condition has been a serious one, but the underlying pathology had been recognised and treated. Nature had determined that during this time energy was drained from her. It was not the result of neglect or mismanagement. But I knew what he was getting at. Her course had been punctuated by episodes of acute deterioration, and procedures had been done on an urgent basis. Several consultants had been involved, several teams, comprising – what, 20 doctors? Onward plans had been made as she was discharged from each episode. Her general practitioner, kept up to date with cryptic discharge summaries, had observed with a careful but non-interventional eye.

I told them the story of her illness, as I understood it. A nine-month saga. To catch up, to provide a sense of continuity in respect of the whole person, required careful explanation. As I explained what had led to what and why, the patient's expression lightened and reminded me of the pupil who suddenly begins to understand a principle of mathematics or chemistry. It all began to make sense.

She left the room looking and sounding better. I had done nothing physically significant.

The reason I asked – or challenged – her husband as to what he meant about a 'whole person' was because I thought her treatment had been good. It was thorough, timely and appropriate. Yet for some reason it has not been satisfactory. True, she was not as well as she or her family expected her to be at this point, but the future was bound to see a gradual improvement. What more could have been done?

It struck me that what this patient and her family needed was not a minute assessment of each symptom, nor more frequent clinical reviews, but a degree of confidence that there was a guiding hand behind the arrangements that had been made. She felt like a pinball, shunted this way and that by unplanned events and opaque decisions. I knew, having read the correspondence with a better understanding of why each step had been taken, that there was a sensible guiding hand. Yet that hand was invisible to the patient, despite the name of the primary consultant being clearly visible on documents and procedure notes. The presence of a central pivot and controlling mind had not been made manifest through clear and measured communication.

What she needed, I concluded, was a more confident perception of where she and her body stood in the natural history of the disease that had afflicted her. If she could visualise better how her symptoms related to the diagnosis on her papers, she would feel less of a wanderer in the unfamiliar territory of illness.

Is it a luxury, to be told in plain terms what is going on? It would seem so, judging by the number of patients who appear bewildered in the maelstrom of events. I can understand why it happens. For doctors dealing with rapidly developing conditions or emergency situations, the priorities are clear – make a diagnosis, decide and treat. It is medically correct. Then, when the treatment has been completed and the anticipated response has been confirmed, the pressure is off. This would be the time to sit down and describe what has happened. But this recap often does not take place. New and more pressing cases have arrived in the hospital. Sometimes it is the most junior member of team who is left to tell the story and they may not understand all of its elements. They will certainly be unsure how to frame the future. The patient is discharged 'better', safe, but relatively disorientated.

So, I concluded, a 'holistic' approach to medicine is quite easy to deliver. It does not, after all, require the specialist to delve into every symptom or system outside their comfort zones. It does not require them to be the patient's GP (specialists are notoriously quick to deflect non-specialised problems back to primary care without so much as hearing patients out). It may be enough just to explain what is happening and why, where the patient sits in the network of involved teams and processes, and how the guiding hand that is rarely visible does actually exist. This hand is not omnipresent or dedicated solely to one patient. It does not promise to sense and respond to every little change. The guiding hand must make decisions and then pull away for a while to get on with other tasks. While it is away, the patient may need to guide themselves. This is possible, but only if patients have a clear perception of where they stand in the story of their illness.

In the third vignette, I explore how detachment from a patient's condition can transform into something more malign.

iii. *Scene: hospital at night.*

9 PM, and the night shift has started. My raggedy handover list contains many jobs; patients to review, 'sickies' to keep an eye on, a chest drain to perform. At 9.30 PM, the bleep goes off – 'fast' bleep. Not a full crash call, but I need to rush. The night is young, and there is energy in my legs, so I sprint up the stairs. Level 8, turn right, rush into the ward. I see movement behind partially drawn curtains, hear the anxious tones of a nurse. I slip into

the bay and see a young woman fitting. A classic epileptic seizure. Her teeth are rammed together. There is saliva at the corners of her mouth. The muscles of her back spasm rhythmically.

'How long has this been going on for?' I ask.

'Five minutes, we gave rectal diazepam.'

Good. A good start. I look at the oxygen saturation monitor. 98% – excellent. The nursing staff have done a great job; there is an oxygen mask on the patient's face. The eyes are closed. I wait to see if the diazepam will have the desired effect of calming those over-excited, frantically firing neurons. But it goes on.

'Give another,' I say. 'Let's give it intravenously this time.'

Another five minutes pass. This is getting serious. A more junior doctor comes into the bay. He has a perplexed look about him.

'Do you know this patient?' I say.

'Yes. She's pseudo.'

I pause. 'This is a pseudoseizure?'

'Probably. I think so.'

'How long she been in hospital? How often does she do this?'

'I only met her yesterday. I think this is her third. She's been doing it for years; she's got notes this thick.'

'How long do they usually last?'

'A few minutes, sometimes 20.'

'You keep an eye on her, I want to read the notes.'

I go to the nurses' station and open the 2-inch-thick folder. It contains letters from neurologists, EEG reports, diplomatic language and couched terms. But there is no question, these fits are medically unexplained, psychogenic non-epileptic seizures (PNES). And that's alright. Everybody has problems. I return to the bedside.

'How's it going?'

'I think they're calming down,' says the senior nurse.

And, indeed, the strength of the spasms is reduced. She must be getting tired, I think. I stand over her and look into the taut muscles of her face. She is flushed. I prise open an eyelid, hoping that by doing this she will see me and respond. The eyelid slams shut once I release my finger. I lean close to her ear and talk loudly, 'Susan, Susan, can you hear me?' I know this is not useful. But I want to make a connection with the conscious mind I know is in there. We have been here nearly 25 minutes now, and I don't want to give any more drugs.

'What do we do?' I say to the assembled staff members. But it is a silly question, because I am the most senior person there. I can't leave her, she's seizing. And I know that a reasonable proportion of patients with pseudo-seizures (yes, a pejorative term, but still widely used among non-experts) have a genuine underlying epileptic disorder. What if this is a real seizure? I've been watching it for half an hour now. This could be status epilepticus, which can be lethal. She might need to go to intensive care, to be intubated, to be sedated, paralysed.

There is a groan. The movements settle. It is over. I make a hasty note and move on. So much other stuff to do.

11:45 PM. Fast bleep. Same ward, but I do not expect it to be Susan. It is. The shift is still the right side of midnight, and I am still positive about life. This time I watch for a while and hold off the sedatives. But the saturations are drifting down, and I don't see or hear good inspirations. I am worried that this is a true fit. Saturations are now 85; it is hard to do that voluntarily. But is any of this voluntary? At some level surely. I feel so useless in the face of extreme 'functional' pathology. What experiences, stresses and terrors could result in a young person making themselves have what looks like a genuine epileptic fit?

After 10 minutes I relent, and we give a sedative intravenously. There is a gradual softening, slowing of the twitches. The saturations are good now. Another 20 minutes has passed. I do not have time to hang around while she regains the ability to communicate and talk. I can't offer counselling overnight. I leave.

3 AM. The lowest hour. My brain craves sleep. In fact, I am sleeping, have been for 30 minutes on a couch that smells of sweat and grime laid down over maybe 30 years. It's probably full of fleas. That sleep has been interrupted by doctors from other teams coming in, making coffees, shaking cereal into loud bowls, slamming the fridge, but it is at least a form of rest.

Fast bleep, level 8: all the goodness that was in me has been left trailing in long, harshly lit corridors. I am now operating at a very basic human level. I will do whatever is necessary to preserve life, but little more. Soon I am standing over Susan again. I shout down at her, shout her name, try and shake her out of it. I think I hate her. I don't understand why the experts to whom she's been referred haven't done better, haven't managed her so that she does not come into hospital and put on such a performance, demanding hours of care from nurses and doctors. Somebody has prepared the sedative, but I raise a hand.

'No point.' We watch and wait. I'm tempted to leave the ward, but I know that would be unacceptable. The nurses are rightly worried. How many hours until daylight? Four. So much could happen in that time. Between now and then I might be required to cardiovert someone, insert a central line, perform a lumbar puncture. I can't be here right now. Why is she doing this? I open an eye and stare down into her pupil. I hope she can see me. If she can, she sees an impatient, angry man. A man with smudges under his eyes and not an ounce of kindness. What will it take for me to show kindness now? A real disease. A patient who suffers through no action of their own. Not like Susan. She knows what she is doing.

It settles. She tires. I hope it is the last one. Next time, I won't come to the ward. Nothing bad is going to happen.

After fresh air and bright sunlight had pushed away the fatigue and allowed the real me back in, I considered Susan's plight. In considering her, I considered my reaction to her. The emotion I felt, a very negative emotion, was genuine. I felt like she was wasting my time. But I knew that she had no wish to be in hospital. I knew that the complex mixture of social and medical circumstances that led to her admission were not chosen. I knew also that the last person on earth likely to show kindness in that situation, will probably be the doctor who is asked to see her at 3 in the morning.

The ability of doctors to respond to 'medically unexplained' or 'functional' disease, or 'somatization' disorders, has been the subject of much investigation and discussion. Usually, the challenge is in the outpatient setting, or in the GP surgery. Every branch of medicine has its own set of disorders that cause significant suffering, but for which no physical explanation can be found. Depending on the type of doctor, their mood or their specific interest, a patient may experience anything from a careful exploration of the circumstances to a brush off, along the lines of 'there's nothing physically wrong...' i.e., – cliché alert – it's all in the mind. Except the mind *is* the patient, and if the mind is driving symptoms, the symptoms are no less troublesome. At the same time, few doctors have the time or expertise to really get into the individual patient's psychosocial background.

Finding a middle way, many doctors develop a form of words to explain medically unexplained symptoms in a non-pejorative way. We describe the strong connections between mind and body, the primitive nerves, the gut-based feelings we all experience under stress, the habits our bodies have of developing unwelcome responses to life events... sympathetic, subtle and non-judgmental. Then we may refer to a super-specialist who has the gifts, or the supporting multi-disciplinary team, to alter the way the mind triggers somatic sensations. Because we know we are not the ones who can really help.

In the fourth scene, I try to remember how to row back across the gulf of detachment that fatigue and irritation can cause to grow between doctor and patient.

iv. *Scene: Emergency Department*

After 13 hours of almost constant work, I got home and fell asleep at 11.30 PM. At 1.30 AM, the phone rang. I answered, to hear about a patient vomiting blood in resus. He was jaundiced. This was going to be a variceal bleed, and I had to get back there in a hurry. The thick nausea that accompanies interruption of deep sleep, with the last, hastily eaten meal still heavy in my stomach, brought out the worst in me. I had plans for the following day; I would be useless now. The night was gone. It would take hours to get in, get to theatre, do the endoscopy and get away again. I hated the patient for doing this to me. I imagined him – an alcoholic, no doubt, who had binged and taken another self-induced hit to liver. Now he was suffering the consequences. In the middle of the night.

As I sped down the almost empty motorway and let cold air in to blast away any residual mental fog, I anticipated my attitude. It was going to be business like. No way was I going to be touchy-feely – there was a job to be done: get the patient anaesthetised, look inside, seal the bleeding point, get out, get home. Then sleep. Sleep.

The white-light glare of the resus bay rekindled any neurons that had not been required to drive the car. I read the casualty card notes and glanced across from the doctors' station to the relevant cubicle. The curtain was drawn.

I walked in boldly. He was awake but groaning. There was blood on his chin and in the bowl that he grasped to his chest. He had all the signs of cirrhosis.

'Hi, I'm Dr Berry. What happened?'

'It just started, doctor.'

'Have you had liver problems before?'

'Not like this.'

'But you've been told there's a liver problem.'

'Oh yes, years ago.'

'Due to alcohol?'

'Of course.'

'Any hepatitis infection, anything like that?'

'No.'

'And… the drinking, have you been drinking recently?'

'Yes. Every day…'

Really? – I thought to myself. You know your liver is scarred and shriveled, yet you carry on. I just don't *get it*.

'How much, recently?'

'Two, three bottles a day.'

'Wine? Cider?'

'Wine.'

'Right. Well, I'm sure you're bleeding from a ruptured blood vessel in your gullet, we need to put you to sleep for a bit and do a camera test.'

'OK.'

I presented him with a consent form and muttered about the risks and the benefits. He signed, an uncoordinated scrawl. I walked away, but he had more to say,

'I knew this was going to happen. They told me. Ever since I started drinking, after the accident…' And then he told me why. Why he had taken to alcohol. The industrial injury, the chronic pain, the enforced retirement, the gap… the gap in his life. My tiredness melted away and the focus, on my own discomfort, was re-directed. Just a few words was all it took. Context.

The story. The reasons.

I approached the bedside and spent a little more time telling him what would happen. The possibility that things could go wrong when I was trying to seal the bleeding point, that he might have to stay on ICU, might be transferred for a shunt, might die. He nodded. It wasn't news.

'Got any family?' I asked.

'Yes. But not here.'

In the car on the way home, as dawn nudged its way under the edge of night, I felt good. The job was done. The sense of satisfaction was high. But for that hour after I was woken, I did hate him, in a way. I wished he didn't exist. But that was when I didn't know him. He was a name in a cubicle. At that moment there was no context, and therefore no empathy, only a natural and not unusual reaction to being woken up. It was the *situation* I hated, not the man. Before I arrived, there was no man, only a problem.

Who's interested in the reactions of a grumpy doctor who's getting tired of being on call? You're paid for it! You get a 5% supplement for being available to come in for emergencies. Get over it!

Well, it is important to examine the reaction to fatigue and disturbed sleep, because it is at these times that patients see the worst of us. The veneer (is it just a veneer?) of compassion is often tarnished in the early hours of the morning, or with the hangover of a recent sleepless night still lingering in the system. The trick at such times is to know how to access the human in ourselves. For me, nowadays, such interruptions are rare and anti-social hours are few. Back in the day when I roamed the wards in the early hours, I frequently transformed into a 'technical' doctor, asking closed questions, focusing on defined tasks and having no spare resources with which to make human connections. It is a biological inevitability – we are less human when we are supposed to be in bed. Yet a third of our patients' lives are lived between midnight and 8AM. We have to find a way to be *nice* at those times. How to do this? In the case I describe, it was by imagining a life disrupted by external events, and the undeserved downward slide into addiction. What if that happened to me? A window into another person's unlucky life, mixed with a dash of imagination – two elements that when mixed can produce instant empathy.

In the final scene, I recall how, during one of the busiest phases of my training, patients became no more than a list of tasks.

v. *Scene: hospital cafe*

It was twenty years ago; I was an SHO, three years post-graduation. The week fluctuated in intensity. After my team had been on call, we had over 30 patients under our care. The name of each patient was on my printed list, followed by columns that I would fill with tasks during the ward round. Once the ward round was finished (hopefully, before midday), I would tackle the most urgent jobs, grab some food, then return to the wards to finish the rest. The day would not end until I had drawn a line through each task. Alternatively, I drew a square next to each and filled in half of it, above a diagonal, to indicate that such and such a test had been sent off or such and such a referral made, only filling in the whole box when a result was back or an opinion obtained.

For three days, that list ruled my life. Consultants or registrars decide what jobs need to be done, and the more enthusiastic, defensive or completist they are, the more jobs they will create. But it is patients who are the true source of jobs. Their failing bodies need us to respond, to test and re-test, to image, to discuss with other specialists. So, to control the list, it was vital that the number of patients be reduced. Some would be well enough to go home in a day or two. Some could be moved to another team's ward (or turfed), but only after an argument (see 'Unwanted').

If the next 'take' day arrived without the list having been radically pruned, we were doomed. 30 new plus 4 or 5 old, I could deal with: 30 new plus 15 old, no way. Jobs would be missed, diagnoses would be delayed, referrals overlooked. The team would leave late, maybe not until after 8 PM. The pressure was on every week to 'clear the decks.' Patients were clutter, patients filled my list... patients were in the way.

Wednesday morning. Jake (my house officer) and I sat on stools in the coffee shop overlooking a recently landscaped park. Next day, Thursday, was the 'take' day. The list stood at 12. We were likely to go to over 40; too many. But things had changed overnight. Mr X had been transferred to King's for brain surgery; I scored a black line through his name. Mrs. Y had been taken over by the respiratory team; the pen struck. Mrs. Z had self-discharged because she was so desperate for heroin. 'Shame!' I said. 'I really hope she hasn't got endocarditis, or she'll be back in a few days.' But she was no longer my concern. If she did re-present to ED, the team on take that day would have to look after her. Mr A was at this very minute being readied for transportation to a nursing home. 'Yes! At last!' I said. The pen moved. Four down. Now we were at eight. Things were beginning to look manageable. Just a couple more. My colleague looked out of the window and remembered something.

'Oh, and the lady on _____ ward, Mrs. B, she died overnight. Pneumonia.'

My pen moved.

'Result!'

Jake looked at me.

'Sorry, that was inappropriate.' I added.

I looked at myself. What the hell was happening to me?

Five scenes demonstrating detachment, the absence of kindness, of patience, of empathy, of care. Yet in one scene, a glimpse of the patient's awful life expanded my mind and led me back to a true understanding of why he had wrecked his liver. Detachment happens. Any patient reading this will recognise the picture of an uninterested doctor; it is one of the ways we preserve our skin. Yet, we must maintain the ability to feel, to be touched, to open up, and to understand when it is necessary. Otherwise, we are as cold as the patients who don't make it out alive.

3.5 Sweat

Josiah Jones came to my clinic feeling nervous, but seemingly unaware that everything about him screamed 'cancer!'. A man in late middle age with recent onset jaundice. No pain, just yellow skin. Some loss of weight and appetite, when pressed. I examined him. Yes, there was the swollen gallbladder. Classic combination – Courvoisier's triad. I was on smooth road here. The next steps were a CT scan and then, assuming it showed what I thought it would show, an endoscopy – my speciality, my favourite procedure. I told him that with a stent in the bile duct his jaundice would rapidly improve, and he would soon begin to feel better. It wouldn't treat the tumour, but all the options available would be considered thereafter – surgery, if it looked like it could be removed in its entirety, or chemotherapy. Neither was a lovely prospect, but at least I would be able to do my part.

The scan took place within days. There it was – a tumour the size of a small tangerine in the pancreas, blocking the bile duct. I confirmed a date for the endoscopy with him.

On the morning of the procedure, I was positive, but also careful to explain the risks. The bile duct and pancreas are delicate areas, and you can get complications when you probe them. Bleeding, infection, and pancreatitis, the unpredictable one. Even when the procedure goes 'well', from the doctor's point of view, the pancreas can become inflamed. Occasionally, it goes into meltdown. Very occasionally, patients deteriorate and are transferred to intensive care. Some do not survive.

It was a struggle, getting into his bile duct. It took longer than usual, and I had to insert a stent into the pancreas as well, to protect it from any injury done during my probing. But an hour later the job was done, and the bile was flowing. I was happy.

When he came around from the sedation, I made arrangements for him to be followed up, and returned to my room ready to treat the next patient on the list. After a few more hours in recovery, he was due to go home.

My mobile phone rang. 'Can you prescribe analgesia, Dr B?' I walked around and felt his stomach. Nice and soft. The paracetamol did not work, so I gave an opiate. By teatime, it was clear that Josiah was not going home as planned. A couple of days in hospital were in prospect, not unusual.

Instead of settling over 48 hours as expected, the pain grew worse. A scan confirmed that the pancreas was swollen and inflamed. His lungs began to fill with fluid, and there was no option but to transfer him to the ICU. I was upfront with him – 'You've been very unlucky. This is now severe pancreatitis. But you are relatively young and fit, you will come through this, but it will take longer than anticipated.'

Next day he was attached to more machines, an infusion pump to maintain blood pressure, a haemofiltration machine to replace the kidneys, which had failed. He looked up at me, his eyes wider than before, still fully conscious. There was bruising on his flanks, where blood had leaked from the pancreas which had now largely dissolved in its own digestive juices. He feared for his life. I held a hand, squeezed it, and said,

'You will come through this.' He smiled faintly. Perhaps he was just being polite. The intensive care consultant looked at me doubtfully. What did I truly believe? I still thought that with all we had to offer, all this technology, and my personal experience of having seen many patients leave hospital (albeit three months later) after equally bad cases of pancreatitis, that he *would* make it.

A week later he was dead.

There is acute nausea. There is mental turmoil. There is self-doubt. There is an unwillingness to do the same procedure again, ever. But there are more patients to be seen. You cannot just opt out. I pressed on. During clinics, on the way home, at unpredictable moments his face and voice intruded. I replayed my actions and my words over and over and again. Then, one of my back teeth fell apart and I had to see a dentist. Diagnosis: root canal. I needed it filled. My second canal. Shit. I made the appointment, lay back, and let the dentist do his thing. With my lips stretched by his latex covered hand, I gazed at the ceiling and thought, 'You deserve this. You *deserve* this pain.' It was a crazy, irrational response. I am no saint or selfless martyr, as I have already demonstrated. But I really did think this, gazing up the bright light. That is the trajectory my mind took. Payback time.

Later, I learned that many doctors follow a similar trajectory after 'bad outcomes', and mine was not so different.

'Stuff happens,' as Donald Rumsfeld commented sanguinely after being questioned about the looting that took place following the fall of Baghdad. 'Stuff happens, and it's untidy.'[13] He certainly felt no personal responsibility for the adverse consequences of a military decision that he had been involved in. The looting was a 'complication'.

That is not the typical response among healthcare workers. Dan Walter, in his book *Collateral Damage* (Herrington House, 2010), describes a terrible complication suffered by his wife, and the panic that he perceived in the young doctor who was involved. A novel cardiac ablation catheter was incorrectly deployed by a trainee, resulting in its spiral end becoming entwined in the chordae tendinae of the mitral valve. When the catheter was eventually removed, bits of heart valve tissue could be seen hanging off it. She developed cardiogenic shock and had to have an emergency mitral valve repair. Dan Walter approached his wife's cubicle.

> 'From behind a cubicle, H____ C____ appeared, and with him was a young man in wrinkled and sweat-soaked scrubs, a young man I'd never seen before, who was shaking like a French soldier.'

Walter paints a vivid picture of the second victim – although many would say that the author – the injured patient's spouse – is the true second victim here, the doctor the third. For now, I'll stick with 'second'.

Susan Donnel Scott, working in Colombia, Missouri, described a sequence of emotions and symptoms experienced by healthcare workers who find themselves involved in patient safety incidents:[14]

> (1) chaos and accident response, (2) intrusive reflections, (3) restoring personal integrity, (4) enduring the inquisition, (5) obtaining emotional first aid and (6) moving on.

In the end, the doctor may 'thrive', that is, learn, improve and possibly use their experiences to help others in similar situations. Others carry on, still feeling the harm and perhaps avoiding certain situations, while a third group drops out. The injury to their confidence is too deep.

After Josiah Jones' death, it took weeks for me to reach equilibrium again. And now, writing a book on the subject, you could argue that I am indeed thriving. I am drawing on the 'injury' (to him, to me) to describe what happens, for others to read. The road to equilibrium involved more than simply thinking things through. Progression along that road involved communicating with colleagues, receiving reassurance and *doing* stuff. Being a doctor. Treating people. Restoring my self-image as a healer and not as a source of harm.

We cannot accept our role in these errors with equanimity. It takes something out of us. This is normal human behaviour, surely – regret, guilt. We are now required to express these feelings to those who have been harmed, as per the Duty of Candour, which became law in the UK in 2014. Following a series of healthcare scandals, the barrister Sir Robert Francis[15] described a culture of obfuscation, and this was followed by *'A Promise to Learn... a commitment to act'* by the American safety expert Don Berwick[16]. This enlarged on the idea of transparency, and finally there came specific recommendations from the Royal College of Surgeons which preceded Regulation 20, or 'The Duty of Candour', that is, the duty to be honest and to apologise. From that point onwards, any doctor working in the NHS who caused 'significant harm'[17] had a legal obligation to say sorry and to explain what happened.

3.6 Guilt

Katherine sat in my office with her head down. I was her educational supervisor and I
had to 'deal' with the situation. She had been qualified for two years, and she was a
good doctor. Yet, for some reason, she had prescribed penicillin to a patient who was
allergic to penicillin.

Junior doctors make mistakes, and how they deal with those mistakes is of crucial
importance. In this dialogue, I explore the psychological reaction and coping me-
chanisms of a Foundation Year doctor who has made a drug error, contributing to the
death of a patient. She speaks with her educational supervisor, me.

My office:

'So, what happened?'

'I made a mistake.'

'I heard about it. How are you doing?'

'Awful. I feel awful.'

'Are you worried? About your career?'

'Yes – well, no, not about being in trouble so much. I know there will be an
investigation, but one of my friends did something similar last year...'

'What happened to him?'

'He had to go on a course, pharmacology and prescribing, and he had to be observed doing drug charts for 6 weeks. But he got through it.'

'I can't guarantee it'll be that straightforward this time, but you're right, I don't see
why you should be struck off or anything like that. Not for a one-off error. The irony
is, however many courses you go on, after this you will never prescribe a drug again
without being one hundred percent sure that the dose is right. You'll be paranoid, but
you'll be safer than most of your mates.'

'I don't want to prescribe anything again. I feel sick whenever I see a drug chart
now. I'm avoiding writing any prescriptions.'

'That's not good. We can't have you not functioning properly. But it will get
easier, I promise.'

'You've had this experience?'

'Every single doctor you ever meet will have had this experience. Any doctor
working in acute medicine will know what it feels like to have done harm.'

'And how did you cope?'

'You have to find a way through it. You must be able to see through it, to the other
side. You know you're going to be a doctor, working for years and years probably, so
you have to put it into perspective. But at the same time, you can't ignore the importance of it.'

'That's what's worrying me. I can't see myself doing this forever. It's too painful,
having experiences like this. I know, when I think about it, that Mr Omar would be
out of hospital, now, if I hadn't written that prescription. He was due to go home in
two days! I know that mistakes often have multiple reasons behind them, system
errors, but in this case, it was me, just me. I remember writing it, the word, the
number. I can't handle that, not again.'

'You are handling it now, in a way. You're here, at work, not at home sick, you're
talking about it. You're finding a way through it.'

'But I don't want to be here. You know what I want? I want to be home.'

'That's natural. It's a need for security, for comfort. It's a response to acute stress.'

'And I keep thinking about dropping out. I have this fantasy of running a book-shop, just sitting there, no stress. I walked past one of the cleaners this morning, and I was jealous. I wanted to do her job. No stress. No complications. Simple tasks...'

'I know what you're saying, but it's not real. That cleaner probably has more stress in her life, more persistently, than you do. You are lucky, you have an amazingly satisfying job. You will always be needed, there will always be patients that need to see you. You have been trained to do that job, and I know that fundamentally you enjoy it! I've seen you at work, remember. You are enthusiastic and genuinely in-terested. I've got no doubt that you'll be fine.'

'Patients won't be coming to see me! If I'm not there, there will be another doctor in my place. I'm not indispensable.'

'Of course. Nobody is. But you have the potential to be very good and to be important to your patients, and to the doctors that you in turn will train. The way I think is this – and I know it sounds harsh – but you have a responsibility to get over this setback.'

'Mr Omar isn't going to get over this setback so quickly, is he? He's still in hospital.'

'That's not the way to think about it.'

'Why? Is my career more important than him?'

'Of course not. And his experience will receive its due attention; we will all look at ourselves. Did we train you properly? Was the system for checking prescriptions working? Were the side effects recognised? We will – we have – apologised to his family. It's not going to be trivialised or brushed under the carpet. But is it right that the mistake should result in a potentially excellent doctor leaving medicine? No, it isn't. There would be no doctors left!'

'I feel really uncomfortable with this. It does feel as though we are belittling his memory, focusing on my future.'

'When I was in your position, years ago, I just kept it all in, didn't talk about it. Perhaps there's something to be said for that.'

'I'm a talker, I'm afraid. I must talk. Do you mind?'

'No, of course not. Look, this is how it goes. Or how it went for me. I made a mistake, it doesn't matter what exactly. A patient died. I hated medicine. I didn't want to come in. I avoided similar situations, just like you have been doing. And then, you know what happened?'

'What?'

'Life happened, that's what. By which I mean, the sun rose and the sun set, shifts came and went, patients arrived that needed to be seen, and they kept coming, and I had to see them and treat them. There was no option. And three weeks later I looked back, and thought – shit, I've seen hundreds of patients since I made that mistake, and nothing bad has happened. I felt safe again, in myself. I felt like a safe doctor. That's how it went for me.'

'Riding a bike.'

'Kind of. You have the skills and the knowledge. You have identified something about yourself through this error...the fact that your memory for drug doses is not perfect, and you have learnt from it. Depending on the policy of this Trust, which I don't know, you may have to do some 'remedial' course or programme, and if that's the case, fine, accept it. Penance. But in three weeks, I promise you, the pain you feel now will be a mental bruise. You'll never forget it, but it will fade.'

'Easy as that.'

'Not easy. Because it will happen again. You can't have a career in medicine, especially a practical specialty, or surgery, if you're that way inclined, and not cause harm occasionally. Every invasive procedure has a complication rate, by their very nature. The chance that you will be the one who *never* has a complication is infinitesimal. So you have to find a way to deal with it. It's going to happen. This is your first time. Your colleagues may experience it this year, next year, in three years' time. Perhaps it's good to go through it now, I don't know. How are you feeling?'

'Just as bad.'

'I can't change that. But time will. We need to talk about something else, by the way.'

'What?'

'The duty of candour.'

'Oh.'

Having determined that she was clearly distressed, I now hit her with another blow. We had another duty to discharge, the duty to say sorry.

3.7 Sorry

Another camera test into the bile ducts. I had been trying to rule out a small cancer with a tiny camera fed into the narrow duct over a two metre long wire. After the procedure he complained of pain. I arranged a scan. There was fluid in his abdomen, surrounding his bowel, pooling at the edges. It was far too much for his own body to have suddenly generated. The explanation was obvious. I pushed the wire in so hard it ruptured the side wall, and all the water that I had pumped through the camera's flushing channel to maintain a clear view had leaked out into his abdominal cavity. It would be infected. It might lead to peritonitis. I had screwed up.

Once I had made the arrangements to keep him safe and called the people who needed to be called, I knew what I had to do. I had to say sorry.

Saying sorry isn't always easy, especially you are feeling sorry for yourself.

'I'm sorry.' I rehearsed it in the mirrored elevator. Exactly what sort of 'sorry' was I preparing to say, I asked myself. Sorry I accidentally perforated your bile duct. Yes, I am sorry. I wish I hadn't. It has caused you pain and trouble (because now I need to take you back to theatre, to close it off with a stent). I am sorry that, on this occasion, I appear to have misjudged the tolerance of your bowel lining while I pushed the camera around a corner. And when I say 'on this occasion', I mean it. This has not happened to me before. I am good at what I do. I am gentle and rarely make mistakes. Today, I did what I always do... nothing different. But for you, of course, it was the only time. So, when I say I am sorry I mean I am sorry for your situation – which is bad – but I am not really apologising for having done something 'wrong'. Yes, clearly something went wrong – but I do wonder, perhaps, if your bile was uncommonly fragile or kinked. Not your fault, obviously, we are all made the way we are made. But maybe not all mine either. Perhaps it would have happened whoever did the procedure. There is a statistical risk to these procedures. We discussed it, when you signed the consent form. It's not a blame game, you see. I want to mention that, somehow, because by saying sorry I don't want to make it sound as though you have a case against me, should you be so minded. It's not an admission of fault. Yes, in terms of cause and effect, the fault has to be mine, as the sole operator, but I can easily refer to my statistics, my record, my training log... to prove that I am no cowboy, no dodgy outlier.

The elevator is slowing. Face it, I am overly concerned with myself. This is about your welfare, not mine. You are the one with four new laparoscopy port wounds on your abdomen. So I will come out and say it... But will I mean it? Will I feel remorse? Does apology require remorse? Does 'sorry' require 'sorrow'? Sorrow... that sounds like an emotion too far; nobody died. So remorse – okay, possibly. But clearly, I am not remorseful. So when I say sorry I might sound a bit robotic. No, I am too good a communicator (actor?) to allow that. I will use all my skills. He will believe I am sincere. Sincerity – that slippery beast. Strangely, I have noticed that genuine emotional responses build within me during difficult conversations, when I am faced with a patient and can see the effect of misfortune on their life – the family photo, the illiterate but charming 'Get Well' card from grand-daughter or son – rather than away from the bed, where I think about it only in the abstract. There is a chance I might go dewy-eyed by the bedside, get sucked into a little vortex of regret, and ask for forgiveness. I will be sincere, when I face him.

3.7.1 *Half an Hour Later*

Was a bit clever. I explained what happened, made it very clear that the perforation must have occurred while I was negotiating a scarred area ('you remember, perhaps, I mentioned that this sometimes happens...') and then described how his pain made me suspicious after the procedure, how I requested a priority CT scan, chased the result and called the surgeon, though fortunately, no operation was required. The way I told it, the whole sequence was an example of exemplary emergency management. Then, wrapping it up, I said, 'And I am very sorry this happened to you, I really am...' He did not hear my deflection, into the passive, the neutral, the whatever an expert in grammar would use to explain how I de-personalised it, de-linked the in-cident, the harm, from myself. '...sorry this happened...' Call it word-play, call it sloped shoulders, something stopped me saying 'I am sorry I did this to you.' I don't like myself for it. I feel like I just ticked a box to adhere to a law. The funny thing is, he was so understanding, and so sympathetic to my situation, so caring in fact – he, the injured one – that my eyes did water, in gratitude, to him.

The Royal College of Surgeons' report *'Building a culture of candour – A review of the threshold for the duty of candour and of the incentives for care organisations to be candid'* (RCS, 2014) seeks to define levels of harm that should trigger an approach to patients and relatives and explores how organisations can be encouraged or compelled to develop a culture that facilitates this. It also touches on the realities of the 'post-paternalistic' era and the demonstration of candour in day-to-day practice.

> Modern medicine offers an abundance of hope, but very few absolute cer-
> tainties. One of the comforts (some would say benefits) of paternalism was
> to obscure this lack of certainty for patients. This is no longer sustainable,

and it means that being candid when things go wrong needs to be grounded in being honest about what could go wrong from the start. Better conversations about risk and the potential for harm are essential for fostering a culture of candour....

These words appear to encourage a greater degree of upfront honesty about the risks of healthcare, rather than waiting for mistakes or unavoidable adverse events to happen before 'owning up'. We could, fancifully, call this 'pre-candour'.

Clinical care is inherently risky, and while organisations and individual clinicians must do all they can to minimise those risks, it will never be possible to eliminate them fully.

Finding the balance between upfront honesty and the provision of 'too much information' is a hard task. Not all patients need or want the same depth of information about risk, even if, objectively, they face similar chances of accidental injury or death.

Opportunities to be open about risks begin in the ED or Admission Unit. Here I sometimes find myself explaining that coming into the hospital is never routine, and that being on a ward brings with it physical and psychological risks. Sometimes this is part of the explanation as to why a patient should *not* be admitted. An example would be a young patient with a headache that does not sound suggestive of meningitis or haemorrhage; coming into hospital will not achieve anything, but they may have been led to expect admission to a ward, and may require convincing that it is right *not* to come in. The same might be true of a more elderly patient with a mild chest infection; they are weak and tired, they might benefit from three days in hospital, but if it is not entirely necessary, medically a case may need to be made about why the risks outweigh the advantages. One begins to speak of 'infections' or 'picking up bugs'. Is it appropriate to be negative about hospitals, and their inherent risks?

The 'hospitals are dangerous' mantra is unhelpful, but it is dishonest to portray hospitalisation in a neutral way. Henry Marsh, a (clearly disillusioned and now retired) neurosurgeon, said in an interview that hospitals are,

... like prisons and there's a huge lack of insight into what a ghastly environment they are.[18]

This is depressing, but he has a point. An alert patient admitted to a general ward for more than a few days is likely to witness distress, disability, physical dependency, acute confusion, wandering, incontinence, the ravages of addiction and sadly, death at close quarters. Even with the most attentive and compassionate nursing, these aspects of frailty and illness cannot be hidden from the watchful. Patients of all ages have mentioned to me how eye-opening and challenging the experience of being an in-patient was. It does not seem unreasonable to explain some of these things in advance.

As to the physical dangers of hospitalisation, the degree of detail we should go into varies. Hospital-acquired infections overall are less frequent nowadays (the incidence of the 'superbugs' MRSA and C Diff has fallen dramatically in recent years), but hospital-acquired pneumonia does remain a common development in the frail population. Should we explain this, or quote the incidence? Do elderly patients and their families, who are coping with the news that they are ill and need to be admitted, need to be told that '...by the way, there's a chance you could catch something else as well...'?

A discussion about upfront candour is essentially a discussion about informed consent. In the context of planned procedures, this is clear and simple; we know which risks require explanation, the patient is enabled to understand these risks in relation to the benefits, and they agree or decline. But when we are discussing admission in the context of acute illness, the use of powerful antibiotics or drips that might facilitate the entrance of organisms into the bloodstream, consent seems less relevant. The patient has no real choice about whether to come in or not. They are ill. To compound the stress of the situation by enumerating the additional risks may well be 'too much information'.

The post-paternalistic culture in which we work emphasises that patients are our equals – partners in care – and nothing should be hidden. However, we must surely remain sensitive to the fact that patients are also vulnerable, and may, in certain circumstances, be happy to 'have things done to them' without full and frank discussion. All doctors will recognise the scenario of the patient who has halted them mid-explanation with the phrase, 'Doc, just do what you need to do, OK.'

The key is in modulating the degree of openness according to the patient's condition, its severity, its acuity, and the signals given off by the patient regarding their need for information. This modulation depends on the doctor's ability to understand the context and judge the person in front of them. Perhaps this requirement on the part of the doctor is *itself* paternalistic, as we are once again putting the *doctor's* interpretation centre stage.

Paternalism is always tempting. It makes life simple. As the authors of the RCS report write, *'One of the comforts [...] of paternalism was to obscure this lack of certainty...'* If things go to plan, and nothing goes wrong, the patient who was not been subjected to a conversation about risk will leave the hospital oblivious to the dangers that they faced, and their experience will in retrospect seem serene. If we are to encourage more 'pre-candour', we must be prepared to help our patients understand and accommodate the anxiety that may be engendered. This will require time to talk, time to listen and time to answer. This is the price of candour, and of true partnership in healthcare.

Consider these errors, each of which I have seen committed by others.

A very junior doctor is tabulating her patients' blood results first thing on a Friday morning before the ward round. This is a standard daily task. She finds that *yesterday* a man's potassium was extremely high at 6.9 mmol/L. The blood was taken in the morning, and the result was on the electronic system by the middle of the afternoon, but for one reason or another, the result was not checked, and no action was taken.

The doctor knows that this put the patient at risk of cardiac arrest, and even as she sits at the computer, looking in horror at the number on the screen, she knows that her patient could drop dead any second. She runs onto the main ward and sees from a short distance that a patient is fine. He glances up and sees the concern on her face. She steps forward and says... What should she say?

There has been an error, a significant omission. The patient's life has been put at risk. But the patient is *fine*. No harm has been done. If she chooses not to tell the patient what she is worried about, but quietly rechecks the blood or prescribes some insulin and dextrose, he may never know the danger he was in. The problem will just recede into history. Should she say sorry?

My feeling here is that the Duty of Candour is not invoked because harm was not done. It is a near miss, and you could argue that the event should be recorded on hospital's register of adverse events. But I think the reasonable doctor would tell the patient that she was concerned about a blood test, and should probably come out with it and say 'we checked your potassium yesterday, it was very high, but I'm afraid the result did not get through to the team,' or something like that. There is no denial, but there is no dramatic telling of what might have happened. Or perhaps she should say more, or her consultant should, along the lines of, 'I'm afraid there was a mistake made yesterday. You were at risk of having a heart attack overnight and thankfully that did not happen. We are very sorry... we think we know why it happened, and we have made sure that all results are seen every evening...' That sounds better.

And this?

A registrar inserts a central line into a patient's neck having obtained their written consent. On the list of potential complications, on the consent form, are infection, bleeding, inadvertent cannulation of the artery (as we know from my previous horrendous experience) and pneumothorax (collapsed lung). Two hours after the central line insertion, while the patient is waiting for the check x-ray which has been somewhat delayed, the patient experiences chest pain and breathlessness. He is examined and there is clear evidence of a pneumothorax on the side where the line was inserted. A portable chest x-ray is done straight away and shows a large pneumothorax. A chest drain is inserted as an emergency, the patient symptoms are relieved, but he stays in for 10 days longer than intended.

Was this an error? It was a known complication, certainly, but it was not intended that the sharp needle would pierce the pleura. Whoever pushed the needle pushed it into the wrong place. That sounds like an error. But the patient agreed to have a procedure knowing that this could happen. Is the duty of candour invoked here?

Well, the patient did come to significant harm (an extra procedure, 10 more days in hospital). If I was the doctor I would certainly come back to the patient, when they were feeling better, and explain what happened; but I would explain also that this is not a particularly infrequent problem, hence the reason we take a focused consent. I would probably say sorry, but not as a personal admission of guilt, but more to say that I was sorry for the situation and sorry that it happened to him. I would feel able to maintain this attitude if I felt that I went into the procedure confident that I was well trained and that I had done everything by the book – be it the use of ultrasound or a good track record of successful insertions. If everything was done as well as it could, then you could argue that the complication was not avoidable.

Such a conversation would be an example of openness, transparency and certainly in the spirit of candour, but I'm not sure if it would tick the box for a formal Duty of Candour response from the Trust.

Remember my missed diagnosis in Part I – the man with a heart attack masquerading as septic shock? Should I have said to Mr Collins, 'Sorry, I was treating you wrong the whole night. I missed the diagnosis... because I didn't know enough, I wasn't clever enough'?

Treatments given are often based on diagnoses which are not clear cut. I remember the look on my registrar's face when she recognised my error the next morning.

Disappointment. I was *expected* to have made that diagnosis. But diagnosis is a skill and sometimes an art and cannot always be correct. The point about the duty of candour is to admit *avoidable* error. To avoid this error, I would have had to have been a different person. Assuming I had studied well and maintained my continuing education and was generally up to scratch, nobody could accuse me of slacking. Nevertheless, a gap in my knowledge was revealed that night. I failed to identify an important medical condition.

But we all have gaps in our knowledge. I made a diagnosis based on the data before me, processed that data through the mind of someone educated to the same level as any other doctor in the hospital. Yet I made the wrong diagnosis. Was that avoidable? Maybe, if the doctor on call that night had knowledge of that heart condition. But missing it wasn't so terribly bad, not for someone of my experience. So let it go, put it down to experience. Mr Collins doesn't ever need to know that he was nearly drowned by all the fluid I gave him.

The unimpeachable doctor might want to meet with him and go through things, to *communicate* – to tell the story of what happened and why. This might include describing how patients with cardiogenic shock can sometimes look as though they have severe sepsis, and that this is what happened. The diagnostic 'mistake' is revealed, but not in way that would categorise it as a formal 'medical error'. Perhaps this is splitting hairs or over-thinking the whole issue. Or perhaps I, like many others, don't need to go looking for grief.

There is a wider question here. Should I have been supervised more closely? Why was a very junior doctor allowed to run the resuscitation bay all night without a more experienced doctor checking up on them. Well, this was the 1990s. Things have changed since, there are more consultants milling about, and the duty of candour wasn't even a twinkle in the Health Secretary's eye.

What of Katherine, the SHO who gave penicillin to the allergic patient?

When she was called in by her educational supervisor (me), the circumstances behind the mistake and prescription were explored. It was probably just a consequence of a doctor being in a hurry. She admitted to that and said she could not even recall looking at the front of the drug chart for the list of allergies. We agreed that the harm must be explained to the patient, and that the duty of candour required her (or us, as a team) to apologise, to explain how it happened and how we would try to stop this in the future. There was no question of failing to admit that an error occurred, because it was obvious. The question was *how* to apologise.

Katherine decided that she must do this herself, under supervision; she felt morally obligated to initiate the conversation. She wondered, as the time scheduled for the meeting with the patient drew near, what she would say. Would she cry? Katherine certainly came close to crying on the day itself. She was horrified with herself. She wanted to give up medicine. She had nearly killed someone who had come in for a completely curable disease.

It depends on the patient's attitude. Sometimes they feel sorry for a clearly regretful or distraught doctor, and they wish to comfort them. Sometimes they, or their relatives, appear to be burning with anger and resentment; they want someone – you – to pay a price. Katherine planned to say sorry straightaway. Then she would explain how it happened. She couldn't make it sound like she was blaming the hospital for keeping her busy. She couldn't suggest she was rushing. She would just have to say that for those few moments she did not pay enough attention during an important task. And then, well, the conversation would go in the direction the conversation wanted to go. However clear your plan, you cannot predict how others will respond.

What I take home from these cases is that the formal process of applying the duty of candour may not be well suited to the wide spectrum of everyday medical error and the many grey areas that exist. The message that I take away is that we must develop the habit of explanation, be quick to tell the story of what happened and why, but not to dwell too long on the emotional or moral weight that comes with the concept of apology. If we have made a mistake we must say so, but all errors occur within a context of uncertainty, and without trying to make excuses, it is reasonable to explore mitigating circumstances. We must find a way of displaying candour while preserving the ability to pick ourselves up and deliver care to the next patient.

3.8 Poison

Charlie's a great guy. He does a good job. He's dependable. But on the stairs just now a colleague told me that Charlie had made a mistake over the weekend. He wrote up a new drug chart (a good old-fashioned one made of card, not electronic like many hospitals have these days) but did not realise that the patient had *two*. The second was in pharmacy, as an unusual medication was being dispensed. The first chart had 'run out', i.e., the row of boxes that need to be signed by the nurse dispensing the drugs on the ward had come to an end. Standard task: copy all the medications onto a fresh chart, then put a line through the old one. Laborious, tedious, but vital. Without a new chart, the patient can receive no medications. Transcribe them incorrectly, and the patient gets the wrong drug or the right drug at the wrong dose; either can be dangerous.

Charlie didn't notice that the patient had two charts. The nurse didn't tell him, and the small, ringed mark in the top right-hand corner (½), indicating that this was the first drug chart of two, didn't make an impact. Charlie is a good-natured, good-humoured, helpful young man. He sat at the nurses' station, copied the drugs over, noted that several had been scored through anyway (antibiotic courses that had been completed, pain killers that were no longer required) and asked the nurse looking after the patient if there was anything else.

'Mr Grey is due his insulin; did you write that up too?' she said.

'No. What dose is he on?'

'Insulatard 12 units twice a day I think, and Actrapid before meals. Isn't it on the chart?'

'Nope.'

'Well, his blood sugar is 18, he needs some.'

'Right, no problem.'

Charlie didn't think to ask – why isn't the insulin on here? He wrote it up. The nurse thanked him and gave the long-acting insulin before she went off shift. The second drug chart was returned from the pharmacy an hour later. This was where Mr Grey's insulin was prescribed. At 8.30 PM another nurse saw that the patient's insulin had not been given at teatime (the box was unsigned), and flustering slightly because of the delay, she injected him with it. Mr Grey fell asleep. At 10 PM, when the nurse was due to check his blood pressure and glucose level, Mr Grey could not be roused. A doctor was called. The blood sugar was checked. 1.5 mmol/L. Mr Grey was in a hypogly-caemic coma. The team injected concentrated glucose. Mr Grey woke up. But he is still not himself. A neurologist has reviewed him, and has concluded that there is likely to be some permanent brain damage; it is too early to tell.

As told to me, I can tell that this is a classic medical error. Many factors, several systemic lapses, failures in communication, failures in process. As I ascend the stairs, I can already visualise the changes that must be made: drug charts must *never* be separated; if there are multiple charts there must be a clear indication, perhaps a coloured sticker; doctors must not write up medication unless they can see the ex-pired prescription in front of them. A nurse's word is not enough. Isn't it obvious – I mean, for God's sake, Charlie, how did you *think* Mr Grey had been getting insulin up to this point if there wasn't a second chart?

I need to talk to him. We have a ward round to do first, but then there will be an opportunity.

I ignore the issue until 11.30 AM. Then I ask him to come with me to a quiet area. We get a cup of coffee. 'Chat with coffee' is code for informal discussion. 'Chat without coffee' means someone is in trouble. He is his usual sunny self. He already knows about the insulin. He doesn't seem too cut up about it. Less than I would been at that stage of my career, anyway. Commendably, he has already thought through the various processes, and he has worked out how to reduce to risk of it happening again. I am a little taken aback. He has done what the system-based investigator would do — that is, look not at individuals in order to apportion blame, but at the organisation. I agree, there are some things to fix here, but… I've got to have a word.

I say, 'Charlie, I agree some of the systems here are archaic; an electronic pre-scribing platform will have abolished that risk entirely. But it's going to be years until the majority of hospitals have that. The next one you work in won't, nor the one after; none of the smaller Trusts will. So you have to stay alert, stay paranoid. Now in this case, we can't get round the fact that you wrote up the drug that was given inappropriately….'

'I was *told* to!'

'By the nurse, yes. There was pressure. But insulin, it's very powerful, you have to be really careful with it, very careful indeed. It's better not to have it for a few hours than have too much. Diabetic ketoacidosis takes quite a while to come on, and Mr Grey was type 2, wasn't he? He would have just run a bit hyper until the evening. So if there is *any* doubt, better to say 'Sorry, I need to see the previous prescription myself, check the doses, not that I don't trust you….'' [I do an act to try to lighten the mood, because now Charlie looks a bit disturbed.] 'Look, our nurses are great, they tend to know everything about the patients, especially on that ward, but at the end of the day it's your signature on the drug chart.'

He looks at me quizzically. This has not gone well, for me. I think I'm okay at feedback conversations, but sometimes….

'Will there be an investigation?' he asks.

'Let's see how Mr Grey is. Certainly, we'll to learn from it, so there will be a short investigation in the department; you may be asked to write down something, what you remember from last night, et cetera. Probably better to do that today actually, or tonight, while it's fresh in your mind. We've all done it, more than once. It's how we learn, how we become safer.'

But Charlie does not seem convinced. Our relationship appears to have changed irrevocably. I was the friendly trainer; now I am the voice of discipline. He will address me differently from now on. But it's necessary. Life is not always smooth on the wards. People are harmed. These events are little drops of poison; they enter our discourse and chill our relationships. We must learn to accept the taste. And to be honest, it is better for Charlie to sample it now rather than later, when he is running a ward or a whole team is relying on him.

3.9 Try

Peter Walker died quickly, but there was nothing we could do to save him. His illness was irreversible. I had stayed late to assess him after his arrival. My instructions to the team on duty overnight had been followed. He had received the best care, in my opinion.

My opinion meant nothing when it came to his family's anger.

They sat across from me at a board table, in one of the meeting rooms on the managerial floor. Wife, sister, son. Also, the hospital's legal advisor and my medical manager.

I spoke first. In gentle tones I commiserated, and then explored what they knew of his condition. With their permission, I then explained what had happened and what we had tried to do to save him.

His wife listened, but I could see the tension in her facial muscles. She was preparing herself.

The son asked some sensible questions. He was the pacifier. He knew what was coming. He had heard it already, at home, in the car, over the phone. He knew that his mother was a bomb waiting to explode.

The sister interjected. Like a scout, she probed my defences and revealed the weaker points. Her questions surprised me. Perhaps she had a point. Perhaps, given what I knew about Peter's condition, I should have made different arrangements, liaised with ICU sooner, warned him, and the family more explicitly that death was a possibility. I had not expected him to deteriorate that quickly.

The wife's mouth opened. She was ready.

For 10 minutes she dissected our care (no; *my* care... I was in charge; the team did as I asked... this was about me) and criticised my management. She fed the fire of her indignation with her own words, recirculating the petroleum phrases and explosive accusations.

I listened. I made no attempt to interrupt. I knew this: grief. The angry stage.

Then she overstepped and used the one phrase that has endured in my mind.

'You should have done better; you didn't *try hard enough*....'

I could not let that pass.

My manager glanced at me, his expression the facial equivalent of a flat hand, as though to say, 'Leave it, leave it.'

She spoke on. I dwelt on the phrase. So what are you saying? I wasn't trying? We weren't bothered? We didn't care? Is that what you're saying? Go on, if that's what you really think.

But no. This is grief. Angry grief. She left her husband in my care and he died, quickly. There was no time for a final conversation. He was put on a ventilator in a hurry. She lost her life companion, the father to her children. This... this spite, is understandable.

The fire in my mouth quietened down. My manager said some neutral things. He offered me the right of reply. I returned to the phrase she had used and reflected it back to her. I had to make her understand that we had worked hard, that he had been the focus of all our efforts, our energy, that our motives were good. We *had* tried. Sometimes diseases progress too quickly, they take us unawares. I was sorry. Truly sorry.

But these were just words now.

Usually, when I say sorry, the basic connection between meaning and emotion is preserved, and I do feel sorry. Not this time. I used the words I was meant to use. There was a recording device on the table, its red light flashing minutely; the legal advisor had brought it along, sensing risk. The SD chip would contain all the right words.

The meeting reached an end. I could barely look at the wife. She did not meet my eye. I hated her. I barely knew her. I hated the wife of a man who had died tragically. What did that say of me?

It took all afternoon for me to process this experience.

How can a doctor hate? Because the doctor feels injured. It is natural to dislike to the person who inflicts the injury.

That negativity now spilled over, staining the memory of Peter, the man I had spoken to, examined; the man who seemed to like me. He knew he was gravely ill. He understood. The important relationship was between me and him, not me and his wife. That was extraneous. I did my best. I didn't make any clear mistakes. Not all illnesses can be cured. He knew that. I had told him. But he was no longer there to represent me in front of his family. I had prepared him for the worst, but not them. That was my mistake.

Expectation management.

The wound healed. I put it down to grief.

It was not about me; it was about her. A cliché, perhaps. But true.

3.10 Burst

Individual errors may lead to serious harm, but the scale remains small. Sometimes, doctors are presented with evidence that their whole approach is wrong. Everything they thought was right, is not.

I was a student at the time, in my fourth year. An administrator's spreadsheet had determined that I was to spend six weeks far from the city in which I was based. For the first time, I would see medicine in a district general hospital, or DGH. These serve smaller populations and are smaller in every way, but their doctors must manage any problem that comes through the front door. There are no super-specialised teams, no abundance of technology or state-of-the-art diagnostic aides. In many ways, doctors who work in DGH have more highly developed wits. They must make do with what they have.

I attended an evening educational meeting, sitting at the back and in the shadows. I, alongside five other students on my year, were spectators, nothing more. Our presence was expected, and although a table was reserved in a nearby curry house, there was no question of leaving early. The consultant whose signature we needed to confirm satisfactory progress during the placement was chairing the meeting. He was young and aggressive, and by all accounts brilliant. That was the general opinion. I was scared of him. He had shouted at me on the stairs three days ago; my crime – not knowing the white cell count and CRP, both markers of infections, for a post-operative patient of his. Shocked, I was later counselled by the junior house officer that he thought I *was* the junior house officer. He was not one for knowing names or faces. But he was brilliant and had already developed new techniques in the repair and bypassing of blocked blood vessels.

There were two vascular surgeons at this DGH. The other one was old and slow. Thinking back now, they were caricatures. The young one, working at the leading edge of invention, demanding the best of all who sailed with him; the older one, with deep experience, who knew when *not* to operate, and confronted complex problems with a deliberate and well-rounded style.

Today's meeting was dedicated to an audit of outcomes after emergency surgery on ruptured aortic aneurysms. I had been present at one of these operations, with the more experienced surgeon, Mr Simpson. It had not gone well. The normal aorta is an inch wide, but in some people, especially older men, its wall thins, and it expands to two or three inches. Occasionally, it bursts. Being the body's central and main artery, all the blood that is pumped out the heart passes through it. When it leaks, blood is lost rapidly, and patients can die in minutes. However, the leak sometimes slows as the pressure builds up around it, giving enough time for paramedics to collect the patient, give fluid and deliver them to a surgeon. The operation must be done swiftly and well. Many do not survive it. Other parts of the body can suffer a loss of blood supply, leading to paralysis, dead legs or strokes. Better techniques have been developed now, involving sleek stents that can be inserted via a small incision in the groin, but in those days, there was only one operation. This one.

Mr Simpson cut a line down the centre of the patient's abdomen. A second draw of the scalpel penetrated the blood-filled cavity, and a red tide swelled up and over the edges. Blood fell in a curtain from the operating table, covering Mr Simpson's legs and filling the short, white rubber boots that he was wearing. Both hands were now concealed within the patient's core. He appeared to rummage for a while. His assistant, a registrar, held retractors to keep the bowel out of the way.

'Dammit! Spleen. It'll have to come out.'

He had nicked the spleen, another blood-filled organ that lies on the left side. The next 15 minutes were given over to tying off its blood vessels and pulling it out, a meagre, brown object.

'Right, back to the real operation,' he quipped. The tension in the room dissipated. Things began to go more slowly. Half an hour later, the job was done.

Mr Simpson tore off the gloves, looked over at me and shrugged.

'We'll see.'

I liked him.

The audit was presented by one of the surgical registrars. He had collected and compared outcomes from the same operation over a four-year period. Outcomes included the big one, mortality, and several others including length of time in hospital, the number of blood units transfused, and long-term disability. The first bar chart was projected. My breaths became shallow. Suddenly, I saw where this was going.

Each outcome was presented in a chart comprising two bars: Surgeon A and Surgeon B. Each chart looked the same. Surgeon A's bar was always higher. His patients were more likely to die. His patients stayed longer. His patients needed more blood. More of his patients were discharged with missing legs or stoma bags. I knew who Surgeon A was. We all did.

Mr Simpson was sitting on the front row. He didn't move until the discussion, when he stood to field polite questions from the audience. None of them was personal. Instead, they explored refinements in technique that might be applied more often. A friend of his, another senior consultant, slipped in a contextual comment: Mr Simpson was one of only two surgeons in the hospital who could perform *all* common emergency operations, including craniotomy (drainage of blood from around the brain) and Hartmann's procedure (removal of perforated lower bowel). He was a *general* surgeon, despite his specialisation in the vascular field. The partisan voice did not need to go on, the point was made. He was *useful*. He had saved many patients.

Was this a coup unfolding before us? What was the purpose of this exercise? Where would it lead? We, the students, were not privy to the politics. We left the room quietly when it was clear that the meeting had dissolved, and soon we were gossiping over poppadoms and naan bread. Mr Simpson had taught countless surgical trainees. He was the go-to surgeon whenever a colleague got into trouble. Yes, said another, but who would you want to operate on your dad?

Even those with fathers had no answer to that. Mr Simpson was not as good, that was the bottom line.

I accompanied Mr Simpson to theatre the next day. He did not seem changed. His head was not hanging. He had been through worse. This was his life.

When my six weeks was up, I had seen enough to understand. Mr Simpson was formed by the density and depth of experience gained over 40 years of operating. He was brilliant, in his way, but he was unchangeable. Soon, his era would be buried under the floes of modernity, super-specialisation, keyhole or robotic surgery, interventional radiology... and his practice would become fossilised.

His younger colleague had made a play. It may not have been the first. The end result would be premature retirement. And looking carefully at Mr Simpson as I said goodbye and thank you for having me, I thought I saw an acceptance of that fact in the lines around his eyes.

Mr Simpson hadn't made any mistakes. If he had, the relatives of the patients who had died would have complained, surely. Either that, or other staff members would have blown the whistle – an anaesthetist perhaps, or the thrusting young surgeon. Mr Simpson's patients did less well, but his treatment of them was still within acceptable parameters. If there are parameters, there is variation. The quality of care given to patients who presented with burst aortic aneurysms varied in that DGH, as it does to this day in every hospital. The patient arriving for surgery does not know who they are going to meet; they do not know if the surgeon standing over them is the best, the worst or just average. Should they? No. The system would fall apart. If only the best can be allowed to operate, we would only have, say, 10 percent of the total number of surgeons available. Many patients would die waiting for their operation. An absurd idea.

We must accept variation. The harder question is, how much variation? To answer this, each area of medicine has developed minimum quality standards, below which teams must not drift. If they do, external bodies may arrive to inspect the department and make, or enforce, recommendations. These standards pertain to individuals too. Cardiothoracic surgery is the best example. Outcome data is routinely collected and centrally collated, allowing 'league tables' to be created. These are controversial, because some surgeons accept and operate on sicker patients. They are bound to have more deaths. But the philosophy of count, collect and publish has been maintained. The audit that compared Mr Simpson's results to his colleagues was just a local, early version of this.

The difference between error and acceptable variation can be impossible to define. While that definition is being thrashed out, patients will continue to be treated by an individual who is under scrutiny.

Audit is a powerful tool. At the age of 26, I walked through the lobby of the Bristol Royal Infirmary every morning. I was newly qualified, and proud of getting a job in the big teaching hospital. On the wood-lined wall was a framed chart of the hospital's management structure, with photographs of each individual. At the top of the tree was John Roylance, the chief executive. James Wisheart also featured as a medical director. I knew both names, not because I had met them or worked with them, but because publicity around the deaths of children undergoing heart surgery was growing. There were regular features in the newspapers and on television. This was 1997. Stephen Dorrell, the health secretary, had announced an inquiry earlier in the year. Now it had been reported that Roylance, Wisheart and Janardan Dhasmana (another surgeon) were to face a General Medical Council (GMC) tribunal. The house depicted on the chart in the lobby was collapsing.

As far back as 1988, a newly arrived anaesthetist called Stephen Bolsin had noticed that an admittedly complex operation on babies with congenital heart abnormalities was taking longer than it should. One of his colleagues, another anaesthetist, said that nobody wanted to anaesthetise Wisheart's patients in the afternoon, because they knew they would not get home to their families at a reasonable time.

Bolsin performed a secret audit on Wisheart, comparing death and disability rates among the paediatric cardiac surgeons who performed high risk surgery. The results confirmed his fears. Two operations in particular were associated with outcomes well below the national average. In 1993, he sent the audit to Roylance and to the Department of Health. A DoH official spoke to Roylance and received reassurances that everything was in hand; improvements were being made, and Dhasmana, one of the surgeons, was on a learning curve. But criticism did not let up. A local GP (and established comedian) Dr Phil Hammond, writing as 'MD' for *Private Eye* magazine, kept up the heat in his regular column. In 1994, the DoH asked the BRI to stop performing the 'arterial switch' operation, but the surgical team conferred and decided to proceed with the next planned case, that of 18-month old Joshua Doyle. He died.

A point of crisis had been reached. Bereaved parents formed the Bristol Heart Babies Action Group, seeking to expose problems in the unit. The BRI brought in external assessors, who concluded that it was a 'high risk' centre. Bolsin flew back to

Australia, perceiving that his career in the UK was over. The GMC initiated an investigation, and in 1997, Roylance and Wisheart had been struck off the medical register for serious professional misconduct. Roylance's error was inaction: he had enough evidence to understand that babies were not safe in his unit. Wisheart's error was one of commission; he kept operating in the face of persistently poor outcomes. Dhasmana was not struck off but was barred from operating for three years.

A public inquiry was undertaken, chaired by Professor Ian Kennedy (the same Kennedy who authored a later report into the criminal malpractice of breast surgeon Ian Paterson).[19] Published in 2001, Kennedy's report made many recommendations designed to make the NHS safer, including an exhortation 'to root out unsafe practices and learn from its errors' and 'to create national standards of care.'

The Bristol Heart Scandal is a terribly sad story. In the context of this book, it illustrates how difficult it is to separate the acceptable from the unacceptable. In this case, it took at least 10 years.

3.11 Curve

There is a moment in medical training when you think you are ready to go it alone. The difficulty is deciding when that moment has arrived. Independence, working without supervision, is a watershed moment.

A gastroenterology registrar who believes that she is ready to deal with bleeding ulcers receives a phone call. A patient is bleeding in the ED. She makes arrangements to bring the patient to the endoscopy unit. She decides not to call her consultant because he has said on several occasions that she is ready. He has 'signed her off'. The patient now awaits her; she takes the endoscope and passes it into his mouth. She finds the ulcer quickly and knows what to do. But it is bleeding rapidly, and the views that she obtains are not very clear. She knows what to do. She washes the ulcer, tries to clean the blood away, but still it bleeds. She begins to feel nervous… even more nervous. She asks for a needle with which to inject adrenaline, hoping that this will slow the bleeding down. Then she might see enough to apply some definitive therapy, a clip or thermal coagulation.

She waits for the endoscopy nurse to get things ready and watches the patient. The elderly man is sedated, but his pulse rate continues to climb despite the blood transfusion. The registrar knows that she would rather her supervisor was here. But then she reflects – this is what independence is about. Coming out of your comfort zone, absorbing the stress, dealing with the situation, making the decisions, …enlarging that zone… making yourself better so you can treat the next patient with even greater confidence and skill. But what if that process involves putting this frail man at risk? She readies herself for the next part of the procedure. She knows that if this goes well, she will emerge from that room a better doctor.

She injects the adrenaline and as she had hoped it has a constricting effect on the blood vessels, causing the flow to slow down. Now when she washes the blood away it takes longer to ooze back, and she can see the culprit in the middle. A raw artery that has been eroded by acid. She chooses to use the heater probe and asks the nurse to make it ready. She passes it down the channel of the endoscope until she can see it emerge on the screen. With one hand she controls the wheels on the endoscope to optimise the position, and with the other she presses the heater probe onto the vessel. Then, with her right foot she presses a pedal on the floor and sends electricity into the probe, creating a tiny zone of intense heat until the vessel is 'cooked'. Thinking that she has sealed the artery, she pulls the probe away. But the bleeding is even worse now. She must have torn the wall away. Quickly she calls for a clip, and the nurse passes her the kit. The registrar pulls out the heater probe and quickly, calmly, replaces it with the clip delivery device. Soon she sees the metal jaws, grossly magnified, floating around the field of scarlet on the screen, and although the view is flooding with blood again, she can still glimpse the artery. Before the window of opportunity has passed, she pushes the clip onto the artery and asks the nurse to deploy. The clip closes down on the artery and stops the bleeding immediately. The field clears and she places two more clips above and below. The patient is stable.

'Well done,' says the nurse 'that wasn't easy. You could tackle anything now.'

But I have to tell you, in the manner of Ian McEwan's playful but tragic novel *Atonement* (Jonathan Cape, 2001), it didn't happen in this way.

She continued to wash away the blood, but the view was terrible. She injected adrenaline and it slowed things down, improving the view. Now the time was right to use the heater probe. She placed its tip on the ulcer, right on the vessel that was spurting blood, and pressed the pedal. The heat dissipated into the pool of blood and made little difference. She knew that a clip was the next best thing, but she needed a better view. She readied the clip, and through the other channel of the endoscope she squirted more water. The view improved, and when the time was right, she deployed the clip. For a while she thought that the job was done, she sighed in relief and smiled at the nurse, but 30 seconds later, the bleeding erupted again, and all views were lost. She took out the camera, bleeped another member of staff to come and help look after the patient, and rang a surgeon. He arrived quickly but argued that the patient was too frail to undergo an operation. The registrar argued back, saying that she could do no more with the endoscope. They debated the pros and cons of various other treatments, and in the end agreed that surgery was the only hope. The patient was anaesthetised and in the operating theatre 40 minutes later. The ulcer was located and sealed. But he did badly after the operation and developed a chest infection. He remained on a ventilator and died seven days later.

The registrar described all this to her consultant – me. From the description, he could see no reason for her to blame herself.

'You did fine.' he says, 'You knew when to give up, that's half the skill.' He doubted that his presence would have made much of a difference. But the registrar knew that the patient's greatest chance of survival would have been afforded if he had not gone to surgery, if the most experienced person had been there to treat the ulcer…if she had not proceeded on her own.

As a trainee approaches the top of a learning curve the moment comes when they have to decide if it is safe to go it alone – the cusp. The patient who comes into hospital on that day will have no idea that they represent a significant moment in the career of the doctor who is called to perform their procedure. They will have no idea where they lie on that learning curve, or that they might form a steppingstone to independence and immaturity. This would not matter if their risk of harm was no greater than that of any other patient having the procedure. But it is the result of this risk analysis that forms a perfect example of how we balance individual risks versus societal benefits in medicine.

Dhasmana, one of the BRI heart surgeons referred to in *Burst*, was on a 'learning curve' too. I have no knowledge of his mind-set, but presumably he must have felt that the lessons he learned from babies who died (despite his best surgical intentions) would, in the end, make a better surgeon of him. Later, when he was cruising the long, high, horizontal part of the curve, patients in that region would receive the best care imaginable. But first he had to get there. There is no way around the learning curve. You can be supervised, but at some point you must fly solo.

The Kennedy report into the deaths of children with congenital heart disease at Bristol in the 1980s explored the learning curve. It quoted Mr Julian Dussek, President of the Society of Cardiothoracic Surgeons:

'The inference to be drawn from the phrase "learning curve" in the context of cardio-thoracic surgery is that there is an expected and acceptable excess of patients who will die or be harmed in the early experience of a learner but who would have fared better if they were operated upon by a surgeon who is on the plateau of experience.'

Wisheart, one of the Bristol heart surgeons, told the inquiry:

'I believe that the reality of the learning curve may be illustrated by the evolution of surgery for transposition of the Great Arteries in this country ... in the late 80s and the very early 90s it was generally understood and accepted that when a unit introduced the Arterial Switch operation for neonates, there would initially be a period of disappointing results.'

Dhasmana submitted written evidence:

'The learning curve in a clinical setting is very difficult to define and defend. In any technical field, there are bound to be 'failures', which improve with increased experience. In complex and technically demanding operations like Arterial Switch, failure usually means loss of life, which is totally unacceptable to any surgeon. Unfortunately it occurs. Though it is unacceptable, its inevitability is well recognised ....'

Is it necessary to accept a degree of 'trial and error' when an individual, or a unit, embarks on a new procedure? Patients who have benefited from heart and liver transplants would say yes. Christiaan Barnard's first patient, Louis Washkansky, lived for only 18 days after the first human-to-human heart transplant in 1967. In 1968, 107 transplants were performed in 24 countries, but the results were so poor that many units abandoned the operation. Only later, in the mid-1970s, when approaches to immunosuppression had been refined, were over 60% of transplanted patients surviving beyond a year. Those who succumbed in the early years died on the learning curve, but they consented to surgery, having no other avenue of hope.

The learning curve for liver transplantation was even longer. The American surgeon Tom Starzl performed the first in 1963, but the young girl with an aggressive liver tumour died during the operation. It was not until the 1980s that improved surgical technique, patient selection and immunosuppression combined to result in acceptable survival figures. Those who had died during or soon after surgery truly were 'guinea pigs'. The surgeons involved must have been strong, focused and unwavering in their belief that they would succeed in the end. They were right, and many people have lived full, or near-full lives because of that commitment.

Atul Gawande, the surgeon and medical writer, wrote in his book *Complications: A Surgeon's Notes on an Imperfect Science* (Henry Holt & Co., 2002),

> To fail to adopt new techniques would mean denying patients meaningful medical advances. Yet the perils of the learning curve are inescapable—no less in practice than in residency.

But not all learning curves relate to innovation. When an inexperienced doctor begins to learn an established technique, the ethics are somewhat different. They must be allowed to train, in order to become proficient and serve their community as an independent practitioner in the future.

Following controversial reports coming out of Parkland Memorial Hospital, the primary teaching institution of University of Texas Southwestern Medical school, a Dallas newspaper investigated. This hospital seemed to take a liberal attitude to surgical training, crediting its juniors with autonomy to proceed with many operations unsupervised.

One faculty supervisor who quit in protest said the mainly poor, minority patients of Dallas County's only public hospital had effectively become 'clinical fodder.' Apparently,

> The head of UT Southwestern's general surgery residency program once said it was 'OK for residents to make mistakes' on patients 'even if they could have been avoided with better faculty supervision,' according to notes taken by a faculty surgeon and later included in court records. Tim Doke, UT Southwestern's spokesman, challenged the accuracy of that account. But Anderson has testified that some faculty believed 'that's how people learn,' though he said he disagreed with the philosophy.

In this case, one supervisor became uncomfortable and complained after he was called into a gall bladder operation much later, after irreversible damage had been done to the bile duct (just like the surgical registrar I witnessed when I was a medical student).

This controversy crystallises an ethical dilemma in medical training. As the journalists put it, 'There's good for the patient, and there's a societal good. We can't exist as a society without physicians learning on the ground.'

A questionnaire study published in the *BMJ* found that 86% of surgical trainees or young consultants had performed procedures for the first time without direct supervision.[20] This appears to be the reality of medical education. Attempts have been made to resolve the dilemma, another BMJ paper seeking to lay out a framework based on respect for the individual, beneficence and non-maleficence. In their introduction Jagsi and Lehmann explained that

The burdens of medical education are not currently distributed fairly. In one US study, students saw disproportionately high numbers of non-white patients and patients with Medicaid (public insurance for the indigent). Another study found that children of doctor parents were less likely to be seen by trainees than were other children.[21]

Pierre Le Morvan and Barbara Stock, from Department of Philosophy and Religion, in New Jersey and Washington, invoked Immanual Kant when seeking to challenge the perception that patients are guinea pigs.[22] They proposed that patients are treated according to the 'Kantian ideal' that one should always treat them as ends in themselves, and never only as a means to another end (i.e., the training of doctors). Their main recommendations are very sensible, developing medical simulation models, enhancing supervision by fully trained consultants and, lastly, changing expectations.

Regarding expectations, if the involvement of trainees is taken into account when the statistical outcome from a procedure is calculated, patients waiting for that procedure are not actually being disadvantaged by having it performed by a trainee. This argument does have a whiff of sophistry about it, but I have found myself using it before. As a patient and a parent, I would want the hospital's best qualified person to treat me or my children (although I am probably too polite to demand as much), but as a trainee I often muttered to myself, in response to a patient's underwhelmed expression, 'Look, this is a *training* hospital...either I do this procedure or it's another five hour wait...what will it be?'

I don't think there is a way of truly resolving the Kantian conflict unless our patients accept that it is not possible to always see the most qualified person in the institution. But the deal must be reciprocated by trainees – they must ensure that every single clinical interaction is approached not from the point of view of 'polishing their resume' (as the *Dallas News* article put it), but from the point of view of the patient. The trainee may well be on the cusp, there may be a theoretically increased risk, but if the skills are embedded, if the trainers have given their blessing, if they feel ready on that particular day or night...no more can be asked.

3.12 Judgement

i. A new role. I am to meet with another consultant whose patients have come to harm through not receiving blood thinners while under his care. Blood clots, or venous thromboembolisms (VTE), can lead to sudden cardiac arrest after patients have gone home. The clots start in the deep veins of the leg and become dislodged, travelling up the body, through the heart and into the lungs. If they are too large, the heart stops.

The VTE team had identified a patient who was readmitted to the hospital two weeks after a major operation on their bowel. The drug chart showed that for five days, Mrs. Barbara Ewell had not received blood thinning injections, and there didn't seem to be a reasonable explanation for this. Sure, if she had been bleeding, or if her blood was already thin for some other reason, it would have been acceptable to omit the injection; but in this case, there appeared to be no excuse. The clot was not large enough to kill her, but her oxygen level had fallen critically low, and she had ended up in the ICU.

The surgeon, Mr Baker, walked into the office. He didn't know me. He had been 'invited' up at this time by another member of the VTE team. I introduced myself. I shook his hand. I explained the process, a mandatory one, by which these cases were identified and investigated. His expression was closed. He didn't want to be here.

I chose my words carefully. With the notes and the drug chart in front of us on the desk, I talked him through the days that followed the operation. Did he recall the ward round on 9th June? Did he remember if there was a reason why Mrs. Ewell couldn't have the injections? Or could it have been... an oversight? He explained what needed to be achieved on a ward round, the checks, the many details. I asked if there was a person tasked with checking on this particular detail. Of course, I already knew the true reason. Mr Baker's ward rounds were notoriously rushed. There was barely any time for the trainees to write down what was said or to assimilate his pronouncements. Minor details like blood thinners would be left to his registrar to keep an eye on.

So, I suggested a more structured approach. I described how sick Mrs. Ewell had become, and how, despite the *excellent* surgical result, it had nearly all been for nothing; she had nearly died. Mr Baker muttered, 'Good. All done then?' and departed. God, that was hard. Yet I knew that he would approach the next ward round differently. It might only be for a week, perhaps a month. Perhaps, if this intervention was effective, forever. My discomfort was part of the price I had to pay for being interested in safety. I was no martyr, and no martinet either. The job had to be done. The effort would be appreciated elsewhere; hey, it might even help me obtain a clinical excellence award.[23]

There was another part in the price to consider. Mr Baker was a colleague. Now, he didn't like me. It was quite likely that one day I would need to call on him for help. In my business, down in the guts and bile ducts, and with my history of doing occasional damage (no more than anyone else), I relied on surgeons to fix things that I could not fix them myself. If Mr Baker was on call when I picked up the phone, the conversation could be frosty. Perhaps he would respond a little more slowly. Perhaps he would let me stew in my own anxiety for a few hours. But no, he was a good surgeon, and professional. I had no need to fear such childish retribution.

    ii. Middle of the night. 3AM. The darkest hour, when our biorhythms demand rest but our patients' pathologies refuse to quieten down. I was reviewing an elderly, unconscious man, Abdul Shah, in a side room. My temper was short, and I muttered to the nurse beside me, 'He's been poisoned, basically.' He was breathing 5 or 6 times a minute, moving barely any air in out of his lungs. Because of this, his carbon dioxide level was high, and he was in a coma. The cause of this was morphine, which had been given every 6 hours for the last three days. Normally, if a patient is in pain and in normal health, that is fine, but Mr Shah was not in normal health. He had kidney failure. It had been worsening over the last week, but little seemed to have been done to diagnose the cause or to correct it. And now the morphine had accumulated to such an extent that he was overdosed. A drug addict lying in a park after too much heroin would have the same clinical features.

The nurse had already called the family, and even though it was the middle of the night, they had come in. I could understand why. Mr Shah was frail, and any further setbacks could prove life threatening. It was unlikely that I would be able to persuade ICU to take him for breathing assistance. All I could do was give naloxone, the antidote to morphine (and heroin), and hope that it woke him up.

In the relatives' room, the family pressed me hard and demanded details. Mr Shah's daughter focused on the kidneys; their failure was new information to her. How? Why? What's been done? Who was in charge over the last few days? I knew the answers to these questions, including the names of the doctors who had been seeing her father, but I refused to divulge. I talked about the 'team', generically. I felt that it could not help the situation to offer up an accountable individual. I feared that in their grief and uncertainty, the family would target one person and focus their anger on him or her. I kept my opinion - that the treatment had been slack - to myself.

> iii. Pancreatic cancer. Again. Maureen was 55 years old. She put the weight loss down to a stomach bug that just wouldn't go away. She went to see her GP when it hadn't improved after 5 weeks, by which time she had lost 4 kg in weight. The GP agreed it was an infection with a long tail and said to come back in a month if it still isn't better. Months pass quickly, and it was 12 weeks before Maureen got round to making the next appointment. By this time her dress size had gone from 16 to 12. Her friends had commented on it. Maureen didn't feel well, and her back was hurting at night in bed now.

I told her the result of the CT scan. 'There is a tumour in the pancreas. It is very close to the blood vessels. We can't say for sure yet without a biopsy, but the most likely cause is cancer. Pancreatic cancer.' Pause. There are many possible reactions. The eyes close, the mouth collapses, the head dips. You know that tears are forming. If they are accompanied, a hand reaches out for support. Or, an immediate coping response. What do we do now? What is the treatment? When will it start? Today: 'Why? Why did it take this long to get a scan? I went to my GP four months ago. Why?'

I am being asked to comment on another doctor's assessment and decision. I am being asked to judge. Do I make excuses for them? Do I agree, and say, 'Yes, you should have been referred as soon as you started to lose weight.'? Or do I try to understand the situation from the GP's point of view - 'Well, at the time I imagine there were no strong indicators or signs of cancer... sometimes people do lose weight temporarily... The GPs I know are very quick to refer on to us if there are *any* concerns about possible cancer...'? Or do I evade and concentrate on the forward plan – the next scan, the visit to the surgeon or the oncologist? What is the point of dwelling on the past, when nothing can be changed?

What drives this instinct to obfuscate? Is there a justification? Surely, in an era of transparency, the patient should know exactly what I am thinking.

It may be a desire to nip a potential complaint in the bud, even when I think a complaint (formal or informal) might be unjustified. If so, am I right to forestall what a more objective person might regard as a necessary corrective?

It may be loyalty to the larger medical community – an instinctive reflex to shield colleagues from criticism, just like in the relatives' room on the ward all those years ago.

Or perhaps it is based on my acceptance that the practice of medicine will always involve variation in knowledge and in quality. Not every biochemical clue will result in the same decision. Each doctor will have developed their own store of knowledge, a unique bank of experiences and memories on which to base their decisions. As long as the decision was not clearly negligent, or so stupid as to warrant immediate correction, we are bound to let borderline or 'sub-optimal' decisions go without making a song and dance. We might hint in a letter back to the GP, or in a comment to a trainee's supervisor, that next time a different decision should be made, and perhaps in that way we reassure ourselves that we have tried to improve the quality of the system. But patients are excluded from this feedback loop. They may go home entirely ignorant of the fact that things *could* have been done better and may not read between the lines of the letter that they are copied into.

Over time I have become more honest about the non-scientific nature of medicine. Sometimes I begin a discussion with the patient with the papers spread out in front of me, or the blood results on the screen, and talk through what may or may not have been going on in their body over the last few years. If I think a spike in a liver enzyme might have been an early signal, which in retrospect was missed, I will tell them, but without loading it with an opinion. It's just a fact. The 'retrospectoscope' can provide a false image of the circumstances that existed years before. Now you are here, let's sort it out. There is no point in opining from the security of the specialist's chair. Misdiagnoses are made there too.

In this way, patients can begin to understand that the narrative of illness may follow numerous detours and diversions before the destination – a firm prognosis, a treatment plan – comes into view. Care is not homogenous, and variability, while sometimes permitting the occasional detour, is an inevitable result of human involvement.

3.13 Fear

I entered the ward expecting a normal, busy day. But the face of the friend who met me by the nurses' station told that something was up.

'What?' I asked.

'Mr Peterson. Bed 19. He's dead.'

I knew Mr Peterson. I had sent him down for a procedure on his liver yesterday. He came back. It seemed to go fine.

'What happened?'

'Overwhelming sepsis. The on-call doctor said it must have been the procedure. He didn't... he didn't get any antibiotic cover.'

My blood froze. Shit. That would have been my job, to write up a prescription for him to receive before he was taken downstairs. I glimpsed the rolled-up sleeve of my consultant through the half open door of the doctors' room. I steadied myself and entered. Fear enveloped me.

Fear is a feature of every trainee doctor's life. In new or particularly challenging roles, it can be a daily occurrence. As the American doctor and writer Danielle Offri observed, our contemporaries in other walks of life rarely feel it:

> I sometimes compare career notes with friends who are in the business world, and I've asked what their worst fear is. It's usually something along the lines of making a financial blunder, screwing up a major project, having

> an investment fall apart, losing a job, disappointing the boss or family, losing money. I have to restrain myself from saying, That's it? That's all you are afraid of? That, of course, is the basic fear in medicine, that we will kill someone, or cause palpable bodily harm.[24]

Is fear limited to the medical profession? That seems unlikely. A policeman or woman on their first shift, or an established detective on hearing that the woman they placated after a complaint of domestic abuse has been found dead; a navy officer taking charge of their first ship, or facing investigation after a near miss on the high sea; a newly qualified barrister presenting their first defence, or explaining to their chambers how a sure-fire win was ultimately lost. All these will feel fear in the workplace. It cannot be restricted to doctors.

The NHS has worked hard to ensure that identifying a locus of blame is not the first instinct after a patient safety incident. Most trainees know this and believe it. Yet, fear remains a common emotion. Despite all the good words about deperso-nalising blame, the facts seem to show otherwise. In a later chapter, we will see how the paediatrician Dr. Hadiza Bawa Garba went through the full gamut of blame, and ultimately was found guilty of Gross Negligence Manslaughter. Despite her success in appealing against the GMCs insistence that she should be struck off forever, the criminal verdict remains in place. The current BMA Chair Dr. Chaand Nagpaul presented the results of a survey suggesting,

> ...nearly 8,000 doctors also found 95 per cent were fearful of making a medical error and more than half feared they would be blamed for problems arising from failures in the system.[25]

Blame then appears to be alive and well, a conclusion backed up by in the *BMJ* with articles such as 'Back to blame'[26] or an editorial from October 2018 which speaks of doctors who are 'fearful' and who:

> ...increasingly work within a culture of litigation and blame, carrying the full burden of accountability...[27]

But I don't think the average doctor's acute anxiety on the ward or in the ED arises from a fear of prosecution. It is probably more instinctive than that. It can afflict the most confident and assured of us, in the most supportive of systems. Danielle Offri again:

> ...fears can easily spiral out of control and overwhelm students and interns. If this happened only rarely, to only those few who entered the medical field with their own pre-existing mental-health conditions, that would be one thing. But the truth is that the fear overwhelms even the most psychologi-cally sound and well-adjusted trainee. At some point, it happens to nearly every single person who travels through the medical training process. If you don't believe me, just ask any doctor you know.

Fear happens when you think you have messed up. Fear is the physiological and psychological sharp end of responsibility. Usually, it passes. In small doses, it may make us more conscientious. Was it fear of reprimand that motivated me to get up early and prepare for ward rounds when I was a surgical House Officer? Or was it a sense of dedication to my patients? It was probably the former, as those patients were barely known to me. Yes, their names were on my list, but I had not performed the operation, I had not diagnosed them in clinic. The skin I had in the game, at this point, was progression. I needed to move through that job without incident, and maybe learn a few useful things along the way.

So perhaps we can accept the concept of 'medicinal' fear; a little dose sufficient to keep you on your toes. All drugs, as we have seen, have a therapeutic window, and in overdose fear does terrible things. I have seen friends and colleagues paralysed by it, so that they no longer respond in a human way to challenge from the person who dolls it out, preferring instead just to roll over. Their torment will not last forever, after all. They will move on soon. I have seen fear lead to genuine breakdowns, or to changes in career. What it does not do, in these doses, is encourage patient safety.

Fear has played a role in our worst health scandals. Don Berwick focused on this in his aforementioned report on patient safety. He says,

> Patient safety problems exist throughout the NHS as with every other health care system in the world.

> NHS staff are not to blame – in the vast majority of cases, it is the systems, procedures, conditions, environment and constraints they face that lead to patient safety problems.

> Fear is toxic to both safety and improvement.

The importance of a 'no blame' culture in the NHS has become axiomatic. It is accepted that the chain of learning that connects adverse healthcare events to improvements in safety is fatally interrupted when incidents are not reported. He recommends,

> To address these issues the system must:
>
> • Recognise with clarity and courage the need for wide systemic change.
> • Abandon blame as a tool and trust the goodwill and good intentions of the staff.

As a doctor who is involved in mortality and morbidity meetings, I often think about the role of blame in learning lessons. At my level, medicine consists of numerous interactions between just two or three kinds of people – patients and doctors/nurses. If a mistake is reported, an assessment is undertaken as to whether that mistake was due to a fault in the system (e.g., poor process, unclear guidelines, bad IT, poor labelling) or a restricted error on behalf of the health care worker. The latter might include mistakes due to a lack of knowledge or a lack of concentration. But what if the lack of concentration is the result of unintelligent rota design or distraction due to an over-burdened system? The spectrum of potential accountability is wide, but whenever an error is identified it is necessary to see at what point on that spectrum the underlying cause lies. Or the blame.

Let's consider Katherine (again), the junior doctor who gave an antibiotic that the patient was allergic to.

The focus of accountability could reasonably fall on one of several points. It could be the doctor not being aware that the antibiotic contained penicillin or not checking that the patient was allergic. For *not bloody thinking*, her exasperated consultant might say to himself, immediately succumbing to the emotional retort that is 'blame'. Or, could it be that Katherine's educators did not emphasise the danger during her training? Perhaps the drug firm should be criticised for releasing an antibiotic with a fancy trade name that obscures its main ingredient? Or is the Trust to blame for not being responsive to the fact that its doctors are routinely over-pressurised at night and are forced to make decisions in a hurry? Or the Department of Health for capping central funding, or the last government for supporting a policy of austerity... or mortgage lenders in America for contributing to the 2007 financial crisis that led to austerity?

This begins to sound absurd, but the point I'm trying to make is that the chain of blame can be a long one. And when you make a mistake, it is natural to look *up* and around for mitigating circumstances.

Now imagine that the junior doctor is brought into his educational supervisor's office (as she was, in fact). It is explained that the patient came to harm because the doctor prescribed the drug to which the patient was *known* to be allergic. *It's my fault*, is how the doctor will feel. But the educational supervisor will be quick to soften the criticism by explaining that there will be a review of systems and more nurse education so that injections are not actually given if it says penicillin allergy on a drug chart, and the Trust will arrange some extra pharmacology teaching for House Officers. Use of the misleading trade name will be banned. The system has *learned*. It's not *your* fault.

Immediately the sense of blame rises from the shoulders of the junior doctor, and it becomes clear that it is not just her problem. Should that doctor walk out of the room with no sense of blame? Well, I can recall most of the mistakes that I have made in my career, and the intense sense of blame and guilt that accompanied them, whether it was mismanaging gentamicin and causing renal failure, missing a cord compression or making a late diagnosis on data that I should have interpreted correctly. It is blame, the sense of personal responsibility, that nagged at my mind and made sure I never made the same mistake again. For this reason, I think individual blame does have a role. I am not alone.

The National Patient Safety Agency (NPSA) states that at least 90% of error can be attributed to system problems or 'honest' errors, while only a small percentage are deemed 'culpable'. This data is largely derived from the aviation industry, where many parallels with healthcare have been identified. But even this presents problems. The 'honest error' is still an error. Just because it is honest (i.e., not intentional or negligent; an error that quite would probably have been committed by a peer in the same combination of circumstances), there is still something to be learned by the *individual*.

The famous psychologist James Reason describes person-based and system-based approaches.[28] He attributes unsafe acts to, aberrant mental processes such as forgetfulness, inattention, poor motivation, carelessness, negligence, and recklessness.

Whereas a system approach accepts that,

humans are fallible and errors are to be expected, even in the best organisations. Errors are seen as consequences rather than causes, having their origins not so much in the perversity of human nature as in 'upstream' systemic factors.

For those of us dealing with error on a day-to-day basis, an approach that tackles individual blame while paying heed to system-wide lessons must be taken. For reporting to be encouraged, blame must not be apportioned in public... for that is where shame develops, and its lethal consequence – inhibition. But in private, as we look at near misses and significant errors, we will sometimes accept that it *really was a silly thing to do*. And we will not hide our concern, nor conceal our disappointment if the error appears to indicate a worrying gap in knowledge, method or attitude. If this is the case, a way must be found to lighten the sense of personal blame by looking up at systemic factors (if present), but without allaying personal discomfort entirely. In this way, we (for it will happen to all of us at some point) will remain alert, and perhaps even a little paranoid, when we enter a similar clinical scenario in the future.

This is all well and good, when we are presented with a complaint or an incident. Someone has already done the hard job of highlighting errors. More challenging still, sometimes, is taking that first step – completing the incident report, or, for larger issues, blowing the whistle.

3.14 Eyeroll

Are those who make the choice to put themselves in responsible positions hard-wired to feel personally culpable for every bad thing that happens? To some extent, yes. Doctors are highly conscientious. Their performance is rigorously monitored and assessed during their studies, and throughout the early years of training. There is always somebody watching. Assessments are routine and frequent. To progress, evidence of satisfactory performance must be accumulated. Negative outcomes, mistakes, might accumulate and amount to 'concern'. It is hard to imagine it any other way. Without such assessments, poor or dangerous doctors could glide under the radar and get 'signed off'.

But it may be even more basic than that. I think it is an enhanced sense of connection between one's own actions and the welfare of the patient. Whatever is happening to them, it's my fault. If I misread an ECG and they go on to have a full-blown heart attack, it's my fault. If I prescribe a drug they are allergic to, it's my fault. If I cut the wrong structure during an operation, it's my fault. If not mine, whose? The patient's, for being ill in the first place? The 'system', for not guiding me to the right answer? My seniors, for not being there to check my work?

No. It was me.

It is in these reflections, I think, that fear is nourished.

Caroline Elton, an occupational psychologist who has counselled many struggling doctors published a book, *Also Human: The Inner Lives of Doctors* (Heinemann, 2018). She describes the chronic, long-term emotional strain – an accumulation of acute stressors. Elton describes vividly the overwhelming sense of helplessness and anxiety felt by a newly qualified doctor on day 1.

> All the time that Hilary had been trying to sort out the desperately ill patient, her bleep had been going off, summoning her to the surgical assessment unit (SAU). As soon as the patient was transferred, she dashed down to the SAU and encountered an extremely angry nurse. 'There are nine patients waiting. Where have you been?'
>
> Before Hilary had the opportunity to explain, the nurse gave a rushed account of each of the nine patients whose names were on the whiteboard. Hilary absorbed almost nothing.
>
> 'Is there another doctor here?' she asked, finding it hard to believe that she was expected to fly solo on the SAU as well as on the ward.
>
> 'Emergency admission. Everyone's in theatre,' was the unwelcome response. The nine names on the whiteboard were swimming in front of Hilary's eyes. She was desperate to know if any of the names were higher priority than the others. 'Could you possibly help me work out who I should see first?' Hilary asked.
>
> 'Figure it out yourself, blue eyes,' the nurse replied.

The author is almost incredulous that it can be that bad. Again, one wonders if any other trainee, in any other walk of life, experiences anything quite so stressful. The scenario, of nine patients all needing attention and nobody around to help prioritise or lend perspective, points again to that sense of personal responsibility. Everything depends on *you.* It is hard to think of another job in which your physical action or mental calculation can immediately improve or worsen another human being's welfare to such a great extent.

How to counter this natural tendency to feel fear?

Firstly, we should ask ourselves if fear should be banished entirely. As a patient, I might prefer my doctor or nurse to feel that sense of risk of trepidation that precedes a significant action. Fear might slow them down; it might make them think twice – is this really the right thing to do? Fear can be a warning that you are drifting beyond your competency, or that you don't quite have enough information. Fear makes you careful.

In her book, Caroline Elton mentions the 'detached concern' that doctors were traditionally trained to adopt. This approach has long had its critics, and Elton suggests that chronic detachment has a more insidious effect on mental well-being than emotional engagement. The unpleasant consequences of detachment have already been explored in this section. If we accept that engagement leads to an enhanced sense of accountability/ responsibility for our patients' outcomes, a logical extension is that fear arising from that sense of responsibility is in fact a natural 'side effect' of being a good doctor.

But fear gnaws at the soul. If it proves disabling, it will do no one any good in the long run. It can take the doctor out of the profession, through the phenomenon of 'burnout'. Burnout is high on the agenda of professional and public debate at present.

The author and doctor Siddhartha Mukherjee wrote on it in *The New York Times*.[29] The article explores resilience to stress and describes several essential dimensions along which a doctor must develop in order to 'survive'. Referencing Victor Frankl (1905–1997, a neurologist and holocaust survivor) and Daniel Pink, author of such books as *Drive: The Surprising Truth About What Motivates Us* (Penguin, 2009), Mukherjee writes:

> What allows some humans to acquire resilience in the face of the most brutal and dehumanizing experiences? Frankl traced the roots of resilience not to success or power but to a sense of purpose and the acquisition of meaning. Later writers, including Daniel Pink, expanded Frankl's concept of meaning along three dimensions: purpose, mastery and autonomy. We acquire resilience when we find purpose in our work. We seek mastery — expertise, skills, commitment and recognition — in our domains. And we need autonomy — independence — in what we do.

Purpose, mastery and autonomy. These things come with experience, but gaining experience will undoubtedly involve error. The challenge then must be to understand that life in medicine will involve periods of acute anxiety in relation to those mistakes, and yes, perhaps even fear, but that unless the decisions or behaviour preceding the events are so far outside the norm as to make them cavalier or irresponsible, these episodes will probably improve us. Such bland reassurances do nothing to make a person feel better in the short term, but support and understanding does ensure that over time, be it days or weeks, the doctor involved gets back on track. Speaking personally, the only time I felt real fear as a trainee was when an error led to a meeting in which it was made very clear to me that I was all on my own.

As a supervisor and trainer, the hard balance, I find, is that of defusing the situation of 'blame' while encouraging the doctor to reflect on what they could (often *should*) have done better. For each of these incidents there will be a degree of personal accountability. That is life in medicine – a career of direct accountability for the welfare of others. Somehow, we must all find a way of carrying this without being broken – and not only that, but also ensure that the equally intense positives are recognised and enjoyed.

It always seemed very sensible to focus on resilience as a 'thing', this ability to 'bounce back from tough times, or even triumph in the face of adversity'. It surely is part of the 'hidden curriculum', as Christopher Horne, David Peters and Faye Gishen refer to it in their *BMJ* article, '*Ensuring our future doctors are resilient'*.[30] Why not have seminars on it; why not encourage trainees to go on courses or listen to podcasts? Why not instruct trainee doctors on how to marshal their inner resources, how to organise their lives, how to handle pressure, criticism and fear of failure? Many senior doctors who have pitched and swerved along their own professional journey will say – yes! I would have appreciated that!

There was a backlash. Or an alternative philosophy. Clare Gerada, a London-based GP and former chair of the Royal College of General Practitioners, writes frequently on the subject.[31] She is spurred in large part by her involvement with the families of doctors who have committed suicide while under formal investigation by the GMC. This tragic group is at the far end of a spectrum, and although their experience must force us to take heed, I am not sure the daily challenges met by trainees are in this league; or perhaps the risk of a catastrophic breakdown is routinely underestimated. There have been enough such tragedies for us all to be on our guard.

The alternative philosophy – my interpretation – is that resilience should not come entirely from within but should grow through mutual support with our peers. In an article *'Doctors need to be supported, not trained in resilience'* (*BMJ*, 2015), Gerada and colleagues explored the foundations of resilience (organisational, individual and cultural factors) and are not impressed by the evidence that 'teaching' resilience is particularly effective. She concluded,

> Although individual factors play a part in improving resilience and training can improve resilience, they do so in only a small way. Larger effects are achieved through creating posts, career structures, and team working to improve job satisfaction and continuity and through building in time to think and reflect for all staff and redressing the current bullying culture of shame and blame.[32]

The endpoint of this alternative philosophy is to dissociate the development of resilience from the particular qualities of the individual. Those on the extreme of the reaction against resilience would propose that culture and systems are directly implicated in cases where doctors lack resilience. In fact, resilience has become something of a dirty word. Perhaps, in a perfect culture, it should not be needed at all. One doctor Tweeted,

> Doctors do not need to be more resilient. In fact, doctors have been too resilient, and that's part of what got us into this situation..... 'resilient' [*exasperated emoji face*] Can't eyeroll enough.

A supportive culture that does not allow blame to be placed on individuals will ensure that no doctor will leave the hospital in a black swirl of self-doubt and assumed culpability. If a patient has been harmed or has died through medical error, the fragile human who was closest to the event, and who appears to be 'implicated', will of course feel fearful and guilty. Most would agree that our culture should ensure that before they leave, they should understand that there is always more to the narrative. The system allowed the mistake to happen; it was poorly designed. We will get through this with you. Don't worry. The main thing is that you bounce back...

Yet, as someone who has both supported younger doctors who were involved in error (or complications) and experienced the sickening realisation that I have myself done harm, I know that however supportive the culture, individuals *do* blame themselves. They take the hit. This may be an inevitable consequence of medicine's tradition: the therapeutic interaction is an intensely personal one. The patient must trust the doctor completely, and doctors must concentrate entirely on delivering the best of themselves – their knowledge, their effort, their instinct. The decision that arises from the moment reflects entirely on the doctor. If it is wrong, doctors will naturally doubt themselves. Even if, on further investigation, the system was at fault for permitting that decision to occur (for example, an electronic prescribing system permits an insulin dose to be duplicated without raising an alert), the doctor will go through a period of hell. They will take the blame, even while their seniors seek to learn system-wide lessons. They will visualise the consequences – the unconscious patient, the terrified family. Then, if they are resilient, they will surface. They will be stronger and better, partly because they will have developed a heightened sense of caution when prescribing potentially dangerous drugs, and partly because they will have learnt that is not really possible to do medicine without occasionally causing harm. Understanding how to deal with that, while avoiding paralysis or endless self-recrimination, is part of resilience.

As a clinical and educational supervisor, I must find a place on the line that runs between two cultural extremes – the 'traditional', blame-centred one in which trainees are expected to 'go home and sort themselves out' and the modern ideal that lifts all hints of personal accountability/responsibility (aka 'blame') from their shoulders. The reality, as ever, must lie somewhere in the middle. The older types who 'suffered a 1-in-2 rota but that's how I learnt my trade' and 'got through the bad times' must accept that younger colleagues will not thrive in the same model. Some will take the pain home, and a very small proportion may develop unhealthy, dark thoughts. In the words of Dr Nishma Malek, a trainee GP writing on the differences between 'Generation Y' trainees and the old guard,

> I can't see the system meaningfully adapting in time. So, if our seniors care to bridge that gap, it can only start with looking within their own circles of influence: in opportunities to invest in meaningful relationships with trainees, in their ability to provide some stability as they're buffeted around, and in their power to encourage and protect their sense of purpose.[33]

Then a new term entered the medical vocabulary -- 'Moral injury'. Professor Andrew Goddard, President of the Royal College of Physicians, headlined with it at the RCP annual conference.

It appears to have come from Simon Talbot (a plastic surgeon) and Wendy Dean (a psychiatrist), who applied observations relating to the stress experienced by soldiers to that experienced by medical staff. The theory is, doctors are torn, and therefore morally injured, by competing 'binds' that cannot be resolved without compromising their values. Just as soldiers who cannot resolve the effects of morally repugnant acts that they have undertaken or witnessed may go on to develop PTSD, so doctors who cannot do their job to a reasonable standard suffer an equivalent syndrome.

Just as the soldier is impelled by duty and discipline to kill (and is morally absolved by their nation's perception of the greater good), he or she still has to overcome the feeling that it is 'not right'. In the same way, just as the 'system' demands that a junior doctor in a poorly staffed hospital may have to leave a deteriorating patient for three hours while they tend to even sicker individuals on another ward, they know it is not right and are injured by the knowledge that the first patient may have suffered needlessly. Yet the greater good is still served. Neither the soldier nor the doctor has the power to change the system; they cannot end the war or flood the hospital with extra doctors. They are employed to do their duty, are naturally (according to Talbot and Dean) a 'hyper-responsible, control-freakish lot' and will always try to make the best of a bad situation.

My question is – are there sufficient similarities between medical and military situations to adopt the term 'moral injury' in place of burnout? Is the frontline of battle anything like the frontline of healthcare? These questions are important, for if we are to accept the term 'moral injury' we must run with the parallels and make very sure that our doctors can be protected, or at least treated.

The term 'moral injury' adds to the impression that doctors are victims. Is this true? Is this healthy? The *BMJ* ran a strong editorial criticising the term 'second victim' i.e., the idea that the psychological suffering experienced by health care workers who are involved in patient safety incidents is deep enough to put them in the same league as the injured patients and families. In it, Melissa Clarkson and colleague from the at the University of Kentucky wrote that being seen as a victim diminishes a sense of responsibility for one's actions, thereby reducing the drive to improve.[34]

Perhaps accepting that doctors are being morally injured will engender a similar feeling, one of passivity, victimhood, powerlessness. However, supporters of the shift to moral injury would say that this is exactly the change of emphasis that is required. Burnout suggests the doctor has failed, and that the response is due to personal factors – maybe weakness or vocational misjudgement – whereas injury suggests that harm has come from the environment and is not doctor-specific. This puts the onus on organisations to improve the environment, not on doctors to dig deeper into their mental resources.

In a *Sunday Times* article, Adam Kay, the author of the aforementioned medical memoir *This Is Going To Hurt,* wrote:

> 'If you want to be a pilot, they'll make you speak to a psychologist. If you want to drive a train, they check you can cope if the worst happens and someone jumps if front of your train...[]... but if you want to be a doctor, nothing.'[35]

Put like this, it is striking. Doctors are dropped into scenes of suffering, yet no provision is made for the injuries that are bound to be sustained to their psyche. Why?

Then Kay writes:

> '...by the very nature of the job, bad days at work outnumber the good.'

This is interesting. Is it a bad day, in medicine, when people get ill and die despite our best efforts? Or is that just 'a day'. After all, in entering medicine, we willingly enter a world of suffering and death. Perhaps it is necessary, before adopting the term 'moral injury', to agree on what separates the 'everyday stress' encountered in an important but high-stakes job from definite injuries. Should we expect doctors (again in the words of Kay) 'to bloody get on with it.' Are those who fall, even temporarily, 'histrionic'? (a term applied to Kay after his exit from medicine).

Consider this recent distressing Tweet from a doctor:

> The man I helplessly watched die via haemoptysis[36] exsanguination over the course of 3 minutes behind an NHS curtain. I'll spare the graphic details. The NHS is still rubbish at supporting its staff. Remember though you can only do your best and you remain human.

This horrible experience, and its damaging effect, did not result from competing binds or a heartless organisational culture. It occurred because of disease and the doctor's proximity to its tragic end stage. Unrecognised, the psychological effect could well contribute to burnout or PTSD-type symptoms. So, I would argue that 'moral injury' does not apply here. Of course, a caring system would make available the appropriate psychological support. An excellent system might not wait for the doctor to present him- or herself but take note of the distressing event and offer support pro-actively.

Who will make the distinction between everyday professional 'stress' and 'distress', and true 'moral injury'? Is it dependent on the situation or the psychological robustness of the individual? Just as one soldier will be unaffected by carnage ('this is the job…'), and another will be appalled, so one doctor will thrive in the semi-chaos of a busy shift ('it's a war zone there… you're fighting fires all night… fix one up, move on to the next… I love it') and another will leave in tears, knowing that they could not deliver the quality of care that they were taught to provide. It is doctor-dependent; we all know that. But this does not make the injury, if we choose to use that term, any less deep.

The forces tearing at doctors are not those you would expect. Talbot and Dean, in their July 2018 STAT news article, hone in on the electronic patient record, which 'distract[s] from patient encounters and fragment[s] care…', on patient satisfaction scores that 'silence physicians from providing unwelcome but necessary advice', and on commercial forces that 'drive providers to refer patients within their own systems, even knowing that doing so will delay care…'. These sound like American problems, but similar issues can be identified in the NHS.

The capacity of the NHS is always behind the demand for its services. It serves best those who have potentially mortal problems who are taken on an express route straight to its technologically impressive and highly focused heart. Those who may have cancer are similarly mainlined through its bureaucracy into clinics, scanners and operating theatres. Others, with benign disease, less visible psychological issues or social needs, may find themselves struggling to get a look in. Doctors and health care workers trying to apply guidelines and protocols that are written to a high standard may find themselves unable to provide 'excellent' care in a timely manner. A sense of perpetual 'sub-optimalism' may set in. The gap between the ideal and achievable becomes established. They stop fighting for the best. They sigh and take paths of least resistance. This is burnout. Or if not full-blown burnout, then a kind of smoulder. It is not failure. It is adaptation to a service that can only spend so much. I'm not sure 'moral injury' describes this situation.

We all see doctors who are knocked this way and that by misfortune, complications, 'bad outcomes', but who carry on, apparently metal-jacketed, who turn up and treat the next patient and the next. Are they different? Are they stronger? Are they better? Are they just hiding their injuries? We must accept variability without making judgements. This is more difficult than it sounds.

People like me, 40-something and older, may have become so used to seeing colleagues disappearing into coffee rooms and crying that we were no longer surprised by it. I often wondered, as a trainee, if lawyers, engineers, dentists etc. at a similar career stage witnessed such distress in the workplace on a weekly basis. Of course not. But such was the regularity that it was easy to shrug and think, 'Well, that's medicine'.

The recent focus on mental health, and its de-stigmatisation, are encouraging developments, but we are still a long way from normalising the articulation of psychological distress. It would take a particularly brave second year doctor to come to a ward round and say to his or her team, 'I'm taking myself down to the Occupational Health 24/7 service, I'm not coping well at the moment...' Can you imagine the looks, the quiet comments in the corridor later on? This sounds facetious, but trust me, as a consultant who tries hard to empathise, I would still find it difficult to process this. Of course, the doctor's distress would be taken seriously and sympathetically, but the courage required of the young doctor would be great, and I'm not sure the systems are yet in place for trainees to voluntarily take themselves off and reveal their injuries.

I see where the term 'moral injury' comes from, but I am uneasy about its derivation and its applicability to all forms of mental exhaustion in doctors. Medicine is not a battlefield, and its practitioners are not employed to harm, degrade or kill the enemy. The opposite, in fact. The moral binds are between competing positive actions, not destructive ones. A term derived from the military arena carries with it many connotations – the flavour of battle, of wounding, or doctors facing patients and their relatives across the lines – when in fact the enemy is not them, but inefficiencies and bureaucracies and, yes, maybe the electronic health record.

Should 16-year-olds who are choosing their A-levels be made aware that being a doctor is now felt to have parallels with going to war? Does the NHS have the ability to support its injured? Or to back-fill the fallen so that those who are left to shuffle along and fill the gap in the front line do not put themselves in even greater danger? If not, why on earth would a keen and clever student volunteer to join up?

If we take on the term 'moral injury', we'd better be prepared to look beneath the Kevlar (woven from conscientiousness, role-modelling, fear of failure and bravado) and treat it without putting others at risk.

4

Infamy: On Judgement and Punishment

Are you entirely comfortable with this?

I'm not.

I have made mistakes. Some were 'soft' (you might say), related to miscommunication or feelings. Patients or relatives may have walked away unimpressed or upset, but at least they did walk away. Other mistakes were far more serious, with concrete consequences in terms of pain or suffering, even death. Yet I swerved formal punishment. Sometimes I punished myself or was punished by my conscience. Under its stern gaze, I reflected on the episode, vowed to do better next time... and moved on. At no point did I contemplate giving it all up. At no point was I hauled in front of the hospital's hierarchy or the GMC. None of my trainers had any fundamental concerns about my competence or insight, and in 2010, 14 years after qualifying as a doctor, I became a consultant. Others have not had it so easy.

Accountability and its consequences become very real when medical error comes to the attention of official agencies beyond the hospital's boundary. The contained cycles of learning, though necessarily unpleasant, are no longer in the control of colleagues or educational supervisors. Blame can escalate; blame can mushroom. Public opinion may be stirred. Headlines may be written. Doctors who fail in the public arena become infamous.

No doctor enters the profession anticipating that they will be referred to the GMC or to the police. But for those who do suffer this misfortune, their professional and personal worlds fall apart. The onus of judgement is moved to a panel of dispassionate experts or to a jury of lay people. In Part IV, I will describe my experience with some of those agencies and comment on two well-known cases concerning alleged gross negligence. Each catastrophe started in environments familiar to us all, and with actions that most doctors will be able to recognise, either in themselves or in those they have observed. But first, I will describe my experiences in the coroner's court.

4.1 Cross

I have been to the coroner's court three times, and it is likely that I will go at least as many times again before I retire. Patients die, and if the family are critical of the care they received, or if the coroner senses that there is more to it than meets the eye, an inquest will be called.

Any doctor meaningfully involved in the patient's care is asked to send in a written account of their actions. Weeks or months later the message comes through, that you will be required to attend on a certain date. However confident you are about your

DOI: 10.1201/9781003189824-4

role, confirmation that you will be questioned comes like an injection of iced water into the veins.

You do your research, your background reading. You prepare to defend yourself.

On the day you may be accompanied by a consultant (if you are still a 'junior') or a member of the hospital's legal team. I was 33 years old at my first inquest, still a trainee, and my consultant came along. The coroner's final verdict would reflect on her department, after all. Before taking a seat, I was reminded, 'Remember, inquests are theoretically public; there may be journalists here.'

I won't describe in detail what had happened to the patient; suffice to say, I performed an invasive investigation and he bled to death. But it was a 'known complication', and the coroner was satisfied that I had performed the procedure carefully; moreover, the procedure was *necessary*. The man would have died if I hadn't done it, because we would never have reached the final diagnosis. '*A known complication of a necessary medical procedure*' was the final verdict. That was what the department wanted. We passed the patient's family in the corridor on the way out. I had spoken to his wife on the ward, once. She looked in my direction but did not make eye contact.

My second inquest was much worse. I found myself defending the actions of several doctors during a night shift when I was not in the hospital myself. Because the patient was 'under me', i.e., my name as the owning consultant was above the head of their bed, the coroner felt it was justifiable to cross-examine me and second guess the doctors' decisions.

I danced around the questions, I defended certain actions, I admitted to a degree of uncertainty over others, and kept replying, 'I wasn't there; this is just supposition'. But the coroner kept at it. My shirt stuck to my chest, my face reddened, but I was engaged now, adrenalised, eloquent if necessary, as she homed in on the critical error. And then she sat back and reminded the court of her earlier words, 'An inquest is an exercise in information gathering; its aim is to allow a confident judgement as to the cause of death. It is not primarily about blame...' My knuckles were white on the beech veneer of the witness stand. I felt like a defendant. Her penetrating questions and forensic approach had not felt like 'information gathering'.

I was asked to attend the inquest because I was *responsible* for the patient. That sense of responsibility is something you must learn to live with as a senior doctor. A visit to the coroner's court reinforces how heavy the burden of responsibility can be. How can you carry on with life outside the hospital if responsibility continues even after you leave the building? How can you ever relax?

One way to deal with it is to understand that responsibility does not equal accountability. What's the difference? The two words are largely synonymous, but the difference probably revolves around the place of blame and the likelihood of being asked to pay a penalty. A doctor can function if they accept that they are responsible, in charge, directing the therapeutic strategy... but not if they are fearful that the blame for failure (assuming that treatment is undertaken in good faith and with appropriate expertise) will arrive at their door.

There is a balance, certainly. One cannot take on a senior position in any organisation or service and be entirely immune to blame, but fear of blame cannot infect every interaction. Yet, for all the personal indemnity[37] that working in the NHS offers, you will still feel vulnerable as the doctor in the spotlight.

The lesson I learned from my visits to the coroner's court is that the need for a named, responsible person as a focus of inquiry is incontrovertible, because relatives of the dead have a right to answers and the record must show how or why people died. If not *you*, as consultant in charge, who else will provide those answers? That is the responsibility, to stand up and explain events that would otherwise remain opaque or dissolve into history. However, you cannot expect to be blamed for everything that happened in a complex system that is the hospital. Blame, if apportioned, will be directed at the organisation for which you work.

So, bruised and sensitised by the experience, I returned to my desk under the realisation that it wasn't about me. It was about the patient and those who had been left behind. I was a source of information and had to be professional enough to give a clear narrative without becoming personally defensive. It was the least I could do. Handling hard questions is a role that must be played in the final, posthumous act of a patient's life.

4.2 Peer

i. I am sitting in a meeting room on the second floor of a grand but fusty Manchester hotel. They use a cleaning compound or air freshener that smells like a combination of talcum powder and nursing home. My team is assembling. Our leader is already present. She is likeable, realistic, experienced. We are here to judge a colleague. He was referred to the GMC on account of multiple concerns. We have interviewed him, his peers (both detractors and supporters), we have analysed 50 sets of clinical notes and recorded examples of satisfactory and unsatisfactory decisions or actions. I think I need glasses, because for the first time during one of these performance reviews, my head is killing me.

When he comes in this morning we will ask a series of clinical questions based on the cases we have reviewed. He should not be surprised by them. He could take copies of the notes home with him last night, if he wished. I really hope he did.

What did he do at home? Did he seclude himself in an office or spare room, to revise? What did he tell his wife and children? They must know he is under investigation. He told us, during the initial interview, that he was well supported. He comes across as calm and confident. That could be the problem: no insight into his failings.

The process has been fair, I think. But then I would say that - I am a part of it.

He answers the questions poorly. My paper soon contains more 'U's (unsatisfactory) than 'S's (satisfactory). Alongside each is a domain of good medical practice and a reason: *knowledge – does not appear to know that albumin is an acute response protein; team working – did not hand over unstable patient to colleague*. It's not my decision how this ends, but I begin to see a pattern. Tomorrow we have the observation of clinical skills. Like a trainee attending a membership examination, he will be asked to enter 12 small rooms, each containing an actor, a short scenario written on a laminated sheet, and perhaps a piece of equipment. The most terrifying is the mannikin, which he will be told is an unconscious patient whom he has found lying in a hospital corridor. He will be expected to resuscitate it effectively. I know he will screw it up. To remain slick at basic life support, let alone advanced life support, you must be doing it for real several times a year. Every month, ideally. The last time this man saw a cardiac arrest was probably 30 years ago. I just hope he's done some revision.

It went as badly as I feared. He put the mask on the mannikin upside-down; he performed compressions as though he was giving a massage in a spa. I feared he was just about to have a cardiac event himself, seeing the sweat gather at his temples. Before we got to that, he had already demonstrated some questionable interpersonal traits, his approach over-paternalistic, his manner curt. Unbelievable really: you'd have thought he would be on his best behavior in this, the ultimate test of competence, this crisis point in his career. I wondered, for a minute or two, if he really *wanted* to succeed.

In the wrap up, we each gave our verdict. Nobody wanted to speak first, so our leader set the scene. She emphasised that this doctor undoubtedly did good work and had done for many years. Yet within that corpus were errors, and they were avoidable. They were not errors of medical fact (though we had uncovered more than a few knowledge gaps), but errors of conduct. Although part of a fleet of colleagues, nurses and therapists, he sailed alone. It was not in his nature to bounce questions around the department or to share diagnostic challenges. He made up his mind and stuck to the conclusion, even if new evidence came to light that was clearly incompatible with it. He worked in an old-fashioned way; not surprising perhaps, given his seniority (a.k.a. age), but he was not interested in changing with the times.

My turn. As is customary, I emphasized some positives. Then, breathing in, I listed my concerns. I shuttered my mind to the picture I had generated of his home, his children, his good intentions, his long career, and focused on the present. If a patient were to enter his clinic room tomorrow with a cancer – say, one of the less obvious ones – what was the likelihood that this doctor would reach the correct diagnosis in time to save the patient? Very small, in my opinion. Therefore, I had to recommend that he enter a period of re-training.

My colleagues agreed. Our leader agreed. She kept her opinion to herself until the end, and I was relieved to hear that my impression matched hers.

I did not have to tell him. The news would come to him in writing.

That was a relief.

ii. She was clearly not cut out to be a doctor. There was no real interest, certainly no passion. She had stuttered from one firm to another since graduating, failing in each role. Her supervisors raised a few concerns, then she moved to the next department. Often, her new consultants had no idea what had gone before; they gave her tasks assuming she was could function at the level of competence that was expected of a bright young woman who had graduated from medical school after five years of hard study. They assumed she had mastered simple things like filling out drug charts and recording the outcome of the daily ward rounds. But she hadn't. And now she was working on my firm.

Our patients tended to be more unstable than those she had looked after previously. Their status could change over an hour; they suffered bleeding, ischaemia, infarction, sepsis, pathological processes that do not tend to respect the daily schedule laid out in her timetable of activities. She was supported by another trainee who was one year her senior, but he had his own responsibilities and could not be at her shoulder every hour of the day. The same could be said for the registrar and the consultant... me. We were not always there to help.

We (myself and other consultant colleagues) saw that she was failing. Wrong doses, missed results, wayward diagnoses. We asked ourselves; is this remediable? Can we train her up? To know this, we had to understand what measures had been taken by others. Her file was given to us. It was two inches thick and amounted to a paper trail of failure. There were near misses, minutes of one-to-one meetings, comments from doctors she had encountered during on-calls ('I haven't worked with her before, but I thought I should highlight the difficulties Dr _____ had during last night's shift in the acute medical unit...'). We quickly agreed that, however much time we gave this doctor, whatever proportion of our energies we dedicated to improving her, we would not succeed. She was in the wrong job.

The option of dropping out had been explored with her by previous supervisors. She would not countenance the idea. This was easy to understand. She had given her youth to medicine. There was only one option. She had to be removed from the profession. Somebody had to refer her to the GMC.

It was not me. The hospital's management structure took care of the formalities. I was asked to provide evidence – that is, a handful of examples of substandard medical care: a prescription written in error, the dose 10 times the maximum safe amount (if it had been given – if the nurse had not had the gumption to question it – the patient would have slipped into a coma and may well have died); a diagnosis so outrageous I could not contort my brain around the deductive processes that must have led to it being written down (perhaps she just guessed). As I typed up these accounts, I experienced conflicting emotions. I felt angered that patients had been placed in her care, innocent, ill people who had paid their taxes and who had no idea that on the day they were wheeled into the ED the bright eyed and presentable young lady who picked up their notes was the embodiment of risk. This should have been dealt with months ago! Simultaneously, my throat tightened. To be a doctor had been her ambition since the age of 17 or earlier. Her parents probably wept with pride on the day of her graduation. She would have entered her first hospital feeling good about herself. *Here I am. A doctor.*

Soon, she would find herself the subject of the GMC's icy attention. Patient safety was its *raison d'être*. Remember that, I told myself. It's not about her; it's about the patient who may develop chest pain tomorrow night and who may find themselves beneath her clueless gaze, pen poised to record a mistaken diagnosis. To be fair, there was little danger of that now, as we had arranged enhanced supervision. All her activities were monitored now. She no longer performed as a qualified doctor, but as a student. Therefore, to put it baldly, there was no point in employing her.

How thoroughly depressing.

The time came for me to attend the hearing, undertaken via a video link. I was asked to read or paraphrase my written statement. Others did the same. A week later, I heard the outcome. She had not attended. She had not arranged representation. She had gone home. She was no longer on the medical register. She had disappeared.

I hoped, and I still hope, that she is happier for it.

4.3 Jack

Hadiza Bawa Garba is a paediatrician. In February 2011, she came in to work as a registrar at Leicester Royal Infirmary. She was in her sixth year of specialty training and had recently returned after a period of maternity leave.

Bawa Garba (I'll use the surname; I don't know her personally) assessed a 6-year-old boy called Jack Adcock. He had Down's syndrome, and at the age of 4½ months had undergone surgery on a hole in the heart. He came to hospital with diarrhoea, vomiting and breathing difficulties. Bawa Garba thought he had gastroenteritis and gave intravenous fluids.

A very high blood lactate level test suggested something more serious, possibly sepsis. The chest x-ray showed signs of pneumonia, but the result was not released until several hours later. Bawa Garba administered fluids but no antibiotics. The hospital's blood result system broke down, and she did not see all the relevant data. The supervising consultant attended a handover meeting where Bawa Garba described Jack's case and mentioned the high lactate level, but she did not ask him for advice; nor did he not volunteer to visit the patient.

Jack's blood lactate level improved. His mother Nicky gave him his usual medication around 7 PM. One of the tablets, enalapril, can have a dramatic effect on blood pressure if the person taking it is acutely unwell. She was accustomed to giving Jack his tablets (even in hospital, where many days of his life had been spent) and was not aware of an earlier instruction that enalapril should be withheld that evening.

At around 9 PM, Jack's heart stopped. A crash call went out. Bawa Garba rushed into the bay and mistook Jake for another boy who had a DNACPR order, so she asked for the resuscitation attempt to be abandoned. Then, realising her error, she rescinded this instruction. Further efforts were made, but a heartbeat could not be restored. Jack had died.

Later, Bawa Garba was investigated by the police and the GMC. The Director of Public Prosecutions saw merit in the case, so it went all the way to the criminal court. Bawa Garba was found guilty of Gross Negligence Manslaughter (GNM), given a 2-year suspended jail sentence and suspended from the medical register. She did not go to prison. The GMC argued that suspension was not enough for a doctor guilty of GNM, and she was struck off. In August 2018, the Court of Appeal overturned this, having considered many extenuating factors, including the following:

- Medical and nursing staff shortages
- Failings by nurses and consultants
- IT system failures which led to abnormal laboratory test results not being highlighted
- Deficiencies in handover
- Issues with accessibility of data at the bedside
- Absence of a mechanism for an automatic consultant review

Jack's death was not all on her. As a doctor, it is easy to look on regretfully, shake your head, mutter the cliché 'there but for the grace of God...' and move on, hoping that you will never be brought into court to defend yourself. But if the reaction to the Bawa Garba case stops there, what *good* has come of it?

The most direct good to come from such a tragedy is improvement in the delivery of acute care to children. Leicester Royal Infirmary learnt quickly, well before the criminal case came to court. Writing in *Private Eye*, 'MD' (Dr Phil Hammond[38]), reported that the hospital reached,

> ...23 recommendations, including that the consultant on-call for emergencies should review all the new admissions in person (something that was already happening in units providing a decent standard of consultant-led care).

But there must be other forms of good, applicable to the wider medical community. Every doctor who followed the progress of the case and felt an emotional response must have come away with a personal point of reflection or lesson that translates to their area.

For me, it was trying to understand the concept of shared responsibility that a medical team has for a patient admitted under its care. This reflection derives from the behaviour (widely criticised and somehow off-limits to all forms of inquiry) of the consultant involved in Jack's Adcock's care. It appears that following Jack's death, Bawa Garba was immediately isolated. Again, in the words of *Private Eye*'s MD:

> ...Dr _____ insisted on seeing Jack's parents without her. Given the parents' sudden change in attitude to Dr Bawa Garba from thankful to extremely hostile, it seems likely that blame for Jack's death was apportioned to her...

It looks as though the consultant took no portion of the burden of blame. He stood apart from the chaos, supervisory but uninvolved. The timeline of the case does not support an immediate crystallisation of blame in the minds of Jack's parents, as it was not until the inquest that they heard, from an expert witness, that their son might still be alive if he had been treated better.

Consider again the mini-hierarchy of a medical team. There is a pyramid, based on experience, knowledge and certification. Each member of the team has a supervisory role over those below them. The consultant is responsible for the way the team functions overall. This is challenging in an environment that does not encourage continuity or team stability, but the line of responsibility still holds. If a patient is admitted under my care and dies unexpectedly, it is I who will be asked to justify the decisions that were made if there is an inquest, even if I never met the patient.

If Bawa Garba's very junior Foundation Year colleague had done something wrong that day, such as failing to communicate a seriously abnormal blood gas result that she or he had been asked to process, would Bawa Garba have felt responsible? Would she have stepped forward and taken some of the flak? To make the question less emotive, let's imagine a different scenario. Would *I* feel responsible if, as a general medical consultant on-call from home, 'my' registrar (who may be someone I barely know), failed utterly to consider or diagnose meningococcal sepsis in a 19-year-old?

It depends on the culture. If it is one where shared responsibility is explicit... then yes, I would feel responsible, I would feel nervous. I would act accordingly.

In such a culture, I would be talking to the registrar, checking-in before I turned the bedside light off, asking 'Is everything OK; is there anyone you're worried about?' In that way, I would get a sense of what is happening; my radar would be attuned to risk and to the strengths or relative weaknesses of the trainee, albeit senior (I was still in this position aged 39), doctor who is running that part of the hospital in my name. This seemingly enlightened and 'team-friendly' approach exists in many places, though as you get more senior there is a tendency to be less involved, or to trust the senior trainees to escalate when they feel the need to – *'a picture of a consultant sitting in chair, waiting for [junior staff] to come and get them'*, as said by the judge in Bawa Garba's trial. Standing back, not involved. And not to blame. It is a balance. A fine one.

In Jack Adcock's case, the consultant was physically close. He sat with Bawa Garba at handover. I still find it hard to understand why his radar did not alarm when he was told that Jack's blood pH was 7.08 (i.e., his blood was *acidic*, evidence of a body under extreme, life-threatening stress). Not being a paediatrician, I have told myself that kids behave differently; they can swing from gravely unwell to stable in a matter of hours. I cannot comment on another specialty. But in the field of adult medicine, I can't imagine hearing that information at handover and not feeling a shiver of risk, of impending danger, impelling me go and see the patient myself, to satisfy myself that the medical management and escalation decision were appropriate. It is data that cannot be unseen, and it draws you into the sphere of shared responsibility.

The culture of shared responsibility presents a potential problem. It could encourage a tendency to cover-up mistakes. If every individual error is dissolved among the many, will anyone ever learn? Yes, if the culture is also just, and can discriminate between different grades of error.

Imagine again the hypothetical registrar who missed meningococcal sepsis, showing a serious lapse of judgement or an unacceptable gap in knowledge. What do I do? My initial instinct is to talk. I complete the morning ward round, take the registrar aside, and ask, 'Tell me about your reasoning here.' Assuming I am appalled, what next? I now need to speak to the parents of the teenager who may be brain-damaged or may lose limbs due to diagnostic and therapeutic delay. Do I go in to explain that there has been an error, avoidable harm... do I perform the duty of candour? Probably not, at this early stage. I talk to the parents about the team, about my role, the registrar's role (initial assessment, early decision–making, diagnostic uncertainty). I explain that things could possibly have been done better, but we need to look into that. Then, later, when more information is revealed, I may have to embark on a painful process of investigation, apology, candour and learning. Perhaps even remediation for the registrar, via their educational supervisor or deanery. And yes, there may be a formal complaint or worse. What I do not do is throw the registrar 'under the bus' (an accusation made to her consultant, her hospital, and the GMC, by many of Bawa Garba's supporters). That early interaction will have made it clear to the family that blame rarely settles in one narrow area. And the same goes for blame's extreme corollary, criminality.

Such an approach can be criticised. Relatives (the true 'second victims') may balk at it. Surely, someone *must* be to blame. I do not lie at the end of the spectrum that refuses to see blame in individuals. The NHS can employ bad doctors, and most consultants will have worked with a few. In the case of Bawa Garba, I do see serious underperformance in the available evidence. In a BBC Panorama (2018) report, she said, 'I was probably slower than I used to be, because I was micromanaging and double-checking everything and second-guessing myself all the time.' But does that justify leading her away from the dock in handcuffs?

Organisational and departmental underperformance clearly played their part in Jack Adcock's death. Eventually, the 'system' recognised this and exonerated Bawa Garba. But not before ruining her life.

It is a picture of the NHS, and of the criminal justice system, at its most disappointing.

The case of Hadiza Bawa Gaba presents other troubling issues around the approach to medical error. Many were concerned that ethnicity had played a role in the decision to pursue her through the courts. That is too large and incendiary a topic for me to explore here, but it is worth noting that since this case, the GMC has looked carefully at its treatment of black and ethnic minority doctors who are referred to it. The second area of concern is the use of written reflections after medical error in court. Trainees have always been encouraged to reflect on patient safety incidents. Such reflections form the basis of this book! However, over the last decade or more those reflections have come to form part of a trainee's portfolio, be it paper-based or (increasingly) electronic. When trainees attend their annual appraisal, the existence of such reflections is checked, and particular examples explored in detail. Bawa Gaba's handwritten reflections, created on the instructions of her supervising consultant, were taken and used by the prosecution. It has been confirmed that the jury did not see this 'training encounter form', nor were they told its contents, but nevertheless it was in the prosecution team's bundle of documents and was read by their expert witnesses. It is likely therefore that her reflections meaningfully influenced the case that they made against her in the GNM trial. There followed, unsurprisingly, a lively debate about the safety of reflections. Dan Furmedge, a medical consultant, published a piece in the *BMJ* with the title, 'Written reflection is dead in the water'. He wrote,

> [trainees] have been left wondering how their intimate thoughts, reflections, and learning might be turned against them in court.[39]

And concluded,

> the revelation that these deeply personal entries may be used as evidence feels like a violation and undermines a process originally designed to promote development. Instead of writing honestly, it is likely that reflections will become watered down and non-controversial, if done at all. Trainees will actively avoid reflecting on mistakes or serious incidents — the very things they have a duty to reflect on and for which reflection is most effective.

The end result would appear to be less honesty, less reflection and less learning. That is the opposite of this book's message, and the opposite of what is needed. It has subsequently been emphasized by the medical schools and training deaneries that anonymised reflections are unlikely to be used as evidence, and that trainees should still be encouraged to do them. The GMC released a reassuring 'Factsheet', explaining that 'we don't ask for reflective notes from doctors in order to investigate a concern' and advising that 'the focus of reflection should be on learning, rather than what has gone wrong or writing in length about what has happened'. The message seems to be – don't write down all the details; don't give away the time, the place or the person; focus on what you will do differently in the future, not on what you did on the day in question. These are subtle points. It is not clear yet if the case of Bawa Gaba has led to a permanent change in reflective behaviour.

4.4 Maw

When I heard about the trial of David Sellu, the colorectal surgeon jailed for contributing to the death of a man, Mr Hughes, from faecal peritonitis, I sighed. Like many doctors, I had come to believe that private hospitals are great for stable and 'elective'[40] patients but are not set up (with exceptions) for those who become acutely unwell. Consultants are largely off site, junior support can be threadbare, and there are fewer facilities. It did not surprise me to hear that the patient had lain in his bed for 14 hours (from the time of Sellu's first examination) waiting for an 'urgent' CT scan, and another 10 hours waiting for emergency urgent surgery. By this time, sepsis had set in and it was too late.

David Sellu's book *Did He Save Lives?* (Sweetcroft, 2019) is his account of the case, and of his time in prison. A sense of injustice runs through it, and the reader comes away awed and a little afraid at the way our criminal justice system can take a man, drag him through hell and then turn around, brush him down and say 'Sorry, old chap, we got that one a bit wrong.'

It is a one-sided account, of course, and there are gaps which any forensically minded reader would like to see filled. It is also a prison memoir, with interesting details that only someone who has done time could know. We learn how to turn used teabags into a plug, the etiquette of bunk-bed prioritisation, and the way prisons incentivise good behaviour. Like other highly educated inmates who have written (from Oscar Wilde to Jonathan Aitken), he describes other prisoners like case histories. A civil man, Sellu had to live with daily profanity. He endured hours of daytime television, preferring David Attenborough programmes to the soaps or 'Homes Under the Hammer'. He reflects on how his colorectal surgical career prepared him for the stench of his cellmates' faeces, passed just yards away from his bunk behind a half-height door. His time behind bars is in no way glamorised.

So, what did happen in the BMI Clementine Churchill? To fill the gaps, I ended up reading transcripts of the original sentencing and the appeal judgement. It is tempting to 're-try' the case in your own mind, but of course my – or any other reader's – opinion is worthless. We were not in court. Nevertheless, to understand how this happened, it is helpful to understand the details.

Mr Hughes developed abdominal pain 5 days after a knee replacement, just before he was due to be discharged. Sellu was asked by a colleague to assess the patient. He saw him after an evening clinic and was suspicious of something serious in the abdomen. There was the suggestion of gas under the diaphragm on an x-ray, a fairly sure sign that something had ruptured or perforated. Sellu requested blood tests and a CT scan. He marked the scan request as 'urgent' but did not push for it to be done overnight. He also asked the junior doctor covering the wards to start antibiotics but did not document this in his written plan. The blood tests were not performed (though the young doctor later told Sellu the results were normal), and the antibiotics were not prescribed.

Next day the hospital worked through its routine CT scans before accommodating Mr Hughes at 11.20 AM, 14 hours after the request. It was reported to show a perforation, as expected. The book suggests there was simply gas in the abdomen, though later it is suggested (through the words of an expert witness), that gas had penetrated through to the region around the major blood vessels ('retroperitoneal air and artery tracking'). An urgent operation was scheduled, but Sellu had to wait until routine lists in the afternoon had finished, and an available anaesthetist had to be secured. He did not exercise the rarely used option of breaking into the routine lists – a sure way to make your colleagues unhappy. Mr Hughes' condition was deteriorating, and his nurses were making phone calls and requesting reviews. The operation started at 10 PM. Mr Hughes was unstable; his blood pressure fell. Sellu found that his liver was irregular, in keeping with cirrhosis, though the CT scan had not shown this. He bled more than expected. After surgery, Mr Hughes was transferred to the ICU, but he died later.

The hospital was quick to conduct an internal root cause analysis. Sellu writes that this was 'frank and hard-hitting in its criticism of many of the hospital's procedures and personnel...' Then, an external agency was commissioned by Duncan Empey, medical director of the hospital group. The investigators were asked 'not only to look into the case of Mr Hughes but to do a full trawl through all my work over the previous years...'. The so called Empey report was highly critical, though we do not read excerpts in this book.

The hospital referred Sellu to the GMC. In October 2010, Sellu attended a hearing run by the Medical Practitioners Tribunal Service (MPTS).[41] They found 'no case to answer', but planned to review the decision after the inquest, which was due to happen just a week later.

It was during the inquest (attended by 500 people, Sellu estimates, a number that is hard to believe) that the surgeon's world fell apart. According to Sellu, a misunderstanding about when he saw the CT scan result led the coroner to suspect him of lying. During questioning the coroner said, 'I am going to interrupt you' and asked Sellu to leave to court. Sellu waited, confused. A manager from the private hospital blanked him in the corridor. Then Sellu's barrister emerged to tell him, 'The coroner is going to refer this case to the police as he suspects a crime has been committed.'

'What crime, and by whom?' replied Sellu. He thought it might be the junior doctor, or the hospital management. But it soon sunk in. It was he, Sellu. It was being alleged that he had committed manslaughter. It would be up to the police and the Crown Prosecution Service to decide.

Later came the police questioning, during which Sellu contradicted things that he had stated to the coroner, leading to an additional charge of perjury. Sellu writes, 'I have since discovered it is best not to commit to an oral interview. Under the stress of the occasion, and unable to consult notes and previous records, a person is liable to make statements that could prove inaccurate.'

The trial began two years later.

Sellu is highly critical of the judge, who in his view (and in the view of the appeal court three years later) did not direct the jury properly. Judge Nicols, in his sentencing, concentrated on two points. First, the antibiotic question:

> Although you did make a record of other elements of your care plan for Mr Hughes in your medical notes, there is no reference to antibiotics. Overall, for whatever reason, I am sure that you omitted to give instructions to the RMO [junior doctor] at any stage to prescribe antibiotics for Mr Hughes.

He was in effect saying that Sellu had lied about asking for antibiotics to be given.

Second, he thought the management of Mr H. was too 'laid back' from start to finish.

> You wanted a CT scan of Mr Hughes' abdomen. That was not unreasonable, but you did not make use of the facility, which was also available at the hospital, to have a scan like this done that same night. Instead you instructed it to be done the following morning with a predictable delay of about 12 hours. On the expert evidence called by the Crown which the jury must have accepted, that was simply far too laid back for someone with a suspected perforated bowel.

Sellu was found guilty (the jury voted 10 to 2) and was sentenced to two and half years in prison.

After reading the book I wanted to know more about why and how he was ultimately exonerated. The Court of Appeal judgement is long, referring to legal precedents as you would expect, but it is interesting to read. In overturning the conviction judges, Leveson, Irwin and Globe were critical of Judge Nicol's handling of the expert witnesses and the jury. Two of the prosecution experts loaded their responses to the court with 'assertions'; to me, they sound like moral judgements: 'very bad practice'; 'no reasonable surgeon'; 'embarked on a bizarrely slow and laidback and inadequate treatment and diagnosis regime which if proposed by a candidate for a basic doctor's examination would result in a fail'; 'recklessness'; 'grossly negligent'; 'grossly incompetent'; 'falling below the level of a reasonable practitioner on multiple occasions'.

The appeal judges said,

> Some of them do provide a yardstick against which the jury could consider whether the criminal test had been met. Others are little more than assertion. How were the jury to assess these opinions on what were, ultimately, legal issues?

> ...there is nothing to suggest the experts provided any explanation as to the terminology of many of their opinions. Further, the jury was given no additional guidance by the judge other than that which we have cited from the summing-up as to expert evidence generally.

...The jury was left on its own to trawl through the differing descriptions, which were adduced in evidence essentially by leading questions, essentially asking whether the behaviour under discussion was or was not gross negligence.

...Furthermore, the judge did not repeat the important direction that what was gross negligence was a matter for them and not the experts.

In the circumstances, we do not believe that Mr Sellu had the benefit of sufficiently detailed directions to the jury in relation to the concept of gross negligence contained within the offence of gross negligence manslaughter.

Another issue was the trial judge's handling of a question asked by the jury before they began deliberations:

Two questions: one, could we please be reminded of what we must or are to be deliberating on (evidence)? Two, are we to be deliberating legalities or are to be judging as human beings, lay people?

Reading this and having sat on a jury in a (crown court) trial lasting 10 days myself, I couldn't help thinking... they were lost! What does this strange question mean? Judge Nicols directed them; the appeal judges were not happy with that direction. He did not, in the appeal court's view, lay out a 'route to verdict'.

David Sellu was a busy surgeon. He ran between his NHS and private hospitals, maintaining commitments on both sites with an energy that I, 25 years younger, can only admire. He dealt with correspondence at home through the evenings and worked weekends. He had seen 4500 patients at the BMI Clementine Churchill during his career there and performed over 300 operations (the book says). He had a very healthy private practice, and presumably he had made a great deal of money from it. Perhaps, running from patient to patient, it was not possible to document everything as thoroughly as he would have wished, or to follow through personally on every detail.

Occasionally, patients deteriorate faster than you can possibly imagine. Sellu's clinical impression of Mr Hughes was that he probably had a bowel perforation, but that he was displaying no signs of peritonitis. He made plans but did not push them. Mr Hughes deteriorated. Looking back, that lack of urgency looked like negligence.

The investigators took the classic approach, looking from the end result backwards, rather than trying to see the situation from 'within the tunnel', i.e., asking themselves if the *context* – the clinical information and resources available at each time point – led to a reasonable decision. Nobody can predict the future. Nobody knew that Mr Hughes had cirrhosis (a factor which contributed significantly to Mr Hughes' death and was accepted as such by the appeal court).

However hard we try to focus on systems, processes and safety nets, in the eyes of the law you, the consultant in charge, are responsible for the care that your patients receive. Blame coalesces around the name over the bed. It was Sellu who failed to negotiate a timely CT scan. It was he who chose not to interrupt the routine operating list schedule. It was in his power to transfer Mr Hughes to the nearby NHS hospital. Reading this book, and remembering Sellu as a benign (perhaps even 'diffident', in his own word) presence at Ealing hospital (where I worked for a year), I wondered, did his manner play a role here?

Would a less 'diffident' surgeon have shown no hesitation in forcing through the CT scan, or breaking into the theatre list? Would a more aggressive surgeon have called up the medical director to complain about the delays, or, after Mr Hughes had died, stormed up to the admin offices and made a scene? Perhaps such attempts to spread responsibility early on would have diverted the attention of the investigators and stopped the subsequent descent into hell.

Finally, Sellu considers the duty of candour, which became law in 2014. A senior doctor makes a mistake. A patient is injured, loses function or dies. The doctor apologises and is transparent about any failings in care. The organisation where he or she works commits to making changes, if required. The investigator's report is shared with the victim, if they want to see it. There are improvements.

A senior judge makes a mistake in directing a jury or handling a witness. A man is found guilty, loses his career and a large chunk of his life. There is no apology to the victim. There is no evidence that the organisation where the judge works is committed to avoiding the same mistake in the future. We are not reassured that the same thing will not happen again tomorrow.

4.5 Whistle

i. Dr White was clearly coming to the end of his career. But he had energy, and always turned up for his ward rounds. Unfortunately, his knowledge was out of date. His ability to examine a patient and confirm or revise a diagnosis remained intact, but his instructions were based on guidance that was 20, maybe 30, years old. So, the team listened to his words, then translated them into a modern medical plan. Most of the drug names were unknown to him. I didn't work with him often, but today we were 'post-take' together. All the patients who had been admitted overnight on the 'take' were reviewed on a long, tiring ward round. I and the other, more junior trainees had been up all night, save a few hours of rest snatched here and there. Dr White was fresh, his jaw freshly shaved, his cologne astringent among our stale shirts and damp armpits.

He listened as we presented each case, he asked the patients one or two confirmatory questions, agreed to our plan, made a few minor adjustments ('always leave something for your consultant to add... it makes them feel needed', somebody once advised me) and then he moved on.

The next patient was a middle-aged man with, unusually for that sex, a serious urine infection. I had reviewed him at 5 AM and he seemed to be responding to the antibiotic. Now, as we walked in at 8.55 AM, he looked awful. His skin was grey, his brow glistened, and the nurse standing by his side was pressing the 'stat' button the blood pressure machine repeatedly, trying to get a reading. As I began to tell the story, its digital display flashed, 105/45. Considering that his usual blood pressure was high at 160/95, this was a big change.

I didn't really want to spend time describing the case. I wanted to push fluid through the cannula; he was on the verge of septic shock.

Quickly I summarised the symptoms, the signs, the blood results and the management plan.

'Agree, UTI.' said Dr White. 'Next patient.'

'Err... I think he looks like he needs a bit of resuscitation,[42] Dr White.'

'What have you given him so far?'

'Two litres of Hartmann's.'

'That should do. Don't want to overload him, do we?'

'But... he's very dilated. And that BP.'

'He looks fine. How are you feeling, Mr Jamieson?' he asked, raising his voice. Mr Jamieson nodded.

'Actually, I was thinking of asking ICU to see him. He might need some norad later, if the BP doesn't go up.'

Dr White paused. 'No. He looks fine.'

I exchanged glances with other members of the team. They were studying their laces, or the movement of cars out on the road.

There were only three or four patients left to see, and we completed the ward round in another twenty minutes.

'Thanks, Dr White!' I said brightly. Then I ran back to Mr Jamieson's ward and into his room. The latest BP was 92 systolic. He hadn't passed urine since he had come into the hospital. His body was gradually shutting down. I squeezed a third litre of fluid into his vein using my hands to apply pressure on the bag and asked my house officer to bleep ICU. By lunchtime, he was in the unit, a central line hanging from his neck, noradrenaline seeping into his bloodstream and causing the blood vessels to constrict, thus boosting his blood pressure and saving his kidneys from failure.

'He's dangerous,' I said to a friend in a quiet corner of the coffee shop

'Yes.' My opinion did not seem very novel.

'So, what has been done about it?'

'The guy's been there for years; he'll be retiring in another couple.' says my friend.

'So?'

'He trained in a different era. Half the diseases and treatments that we see now he didn't even learn about.'

'That's no excuse.'

'What do you expect the Trust to do?'

'Take him off the on-call rota. Patients are being exposed to him every week.'

'And what would that cost? They'd have to employ another consultant.'

'Does it matter?'

'No, of course not. But can you prove that he has actually caused a patient to suffer or die?'

'Well, I've just described a case where that has obviously happened. I can't believe nobody has ever said anything.'

'But you made the right diagnosis and sorted the patient out. No harm. He's surrounded by juniors who know what to do. What do you want to do, whistle blow?'

'I'm tempted to. Who should I talk to?'

'Your educational supervisor. That's who I would go to. Is he friendly, your supervisor?'

'She's a *she*. A surgeon. I'm not sure she would have a strong opinion on the medical detail.'

'It doesn't matter. She doesn't have to. She just has to acknowledge your concern. She'll have an obligation to go up the chain. What about the GMC?'

'What will they do?'

'I've heard there's a hotline they're setting up.'

'You know what I think would happen if I told them?'

'What?'

'I think it would ruin my life.'

'Why?'

'Because for the rest of my time here I would be thinking about what was going to happen.'

'In what way?'

'Well…I'm sure they would be discreet, but they would need evidence from me. I would have to provide reports, or they would have to come down and find them. That would become the focus of my life. Makes me feel ill thinking about it.'

'We had something like this on the ethics station in our exam. If there is a real, imminent risk of patient safety, the answer was easy. You have to re- move the doctor from the clinical environment.'

'Yes, but that was for doctors on drugs, or drunk.'

'What's the difference? A danger is a danger. If you really think he's a danger, then you should go to someone. The medical director or something like that?'

'Didn't you work with him a while back? Didn't you notice anything?'

'Yes, I thought he was crap.'

'And did you go and speak to anybody?'

'No. He wasn't *that* crap.'

'But now you know, having spoken to me, that he is *that* crap. We agree. I'm sure if there were a few others in here we'd all agree. Shouldn't we all do something about it?'

It was not clear to me or my friend that Dr White was a genuine danger. Prior to our arrival in the Trust, just two and half months ago, he had been employed for over 30 years without serious complaint. So why should it come to us, young doctors at the beginning of our careers, to raise the alarm? Surely, if no-one else had detected his deficiencies, it was more likely that *we* were wrong. Perhaps our inexperience had led us to misinterpret the things we had witnessed.

And, after all, did those patients *really* suffer more because of Dr White's decisions? The man with septic shock recovered. Can you really expect con- sultants, who see each patient for 10 minutes after they have already been the hospital for up to 12 hours already, to make every diagnosis, to make no errors? And hadn't Dr White seen another 15 patients on that post a ward round, making the right diagnosis and the right decision for the overwhelming majority?

I did nothing.

ii. In 2014, a junior doctor called Chris Day came to work in an ICU and found himself looking after 15 (some reports say 18) critically ill patients, a job he was not trained to do. He was also responsible for four other wards. Two doctors had called in sick, leaving him isolated. He reported the situation, making a 'protected disclosure' to the Trust and the regional post-graduate education body, blowing the whistle on poor levels of staffing in Queen Elizabeth Hospital (QEH), Woolwich. In doing so, he ruined his career. Health Education England (HEE), the organization responsible for overseeing doctors in training, decided that due to 'conduct' issues, Dr Day should be removed from his training programme. They did not support him in blowing the whistle on poor conditions at QEH, and in fact dissociated themselves from any responsibility for trainees in his position.

> Our position is that Dr Day resigned from his training programme despite HEE staff supporting him and encouraging him to remain on his training programme. We have been very clear all along that we strongly deny that HEE staff caused Dr Day detriment and in fact did what they could to help him which is what we will argue in the tribunal.

They were not his employer, and therefore had no duty of care. This position was finally overturned by the Court of Appeal in May 2017, and one year later, at his final employment tribunal, Dr Day was awarded £55,000 in costs and compensation. For three years, he had sustained himself by working as a locum. Through his persistence, Chris Day established a precedent and forced the establishment to accept that that junior doctors are indeed protected by whistleblowing protections under the Employment Rights Act.

I observed his progress, and asked myself – for all my enthusiasm for safety, for learning from error, would I have the courage to do the same? After all, I had myself worked in critically understaffed departments and wards. I had observed, and accepted, high risk environments. Yet I had done nothing. I had 'buckled down' and got on with it. Perhaps a different me – a braver version – would have stepped up...

It is easier to imagine it vicariously. Let's hear Adam. A brave one...

Adam and I sat in a beer garden. Adam occasionally looked over his shoulder to check who had taken the adjacent table.

'Was it you?' I asked.

'What?'

'Who called the GMC.'

'What did you hear?'

'That someone blew the whistle on A and E.'

'What else did you hear?'

'That it was about staffing levels, lack of support...it *was* you, wasn't it?'

'Why do you think it was me?'

'Because you've been going on about it for ages.'

'That's the point, I guess. I wasn't seeing any changes at all. I was out of ideas.'

'So, did you actually complain first, officially...through proper channels?'

'I told the clinical lead that I thought we were too thin on the ground. Several times.'

'And what did she say?'

'That it "will get better." That "when the deanery sends us more juniors we'll be fine". Mañana, mañana.'

'Did you have examples of poor staffing leading to bad outcomes?'

'How can you get that evidence? We're working on the ground, struggling, we work our arses off to keep the ship afloat; some people die, most don't; how do I know if any particular death is directly related to not enough staff? How do I know if our department has got more deaths or delayed diagnoses that average? I don't have that overview.'

'So how can you justify blowing the whistle? You don't know that the department was actually under-performing.'

'If you follow that line of reasoning, no one would ever stand up and say anything; they will have no confidence in their own opinion. *'I'm just a cog in a machine, I'm not driving the machine'*. To justify NOT saying anything you must have complete faith in the driver. Do I have faith in the driver? I don't know; I don't know the people who run the hospital. All I know is that sometimes it's hell in that department and patients are falling off their chairs in the waiting room.'

'And despite not *knowing*, you made the call. Where did you develop that confidence in yourself?'

'It's not confidence. It didn't come easy. I waited for months and months before making that phone call. Nearly a year in fact. But nothing was changing.'

'It has now.'

'I know.'

'You should feel proud.'

'I don't. I just feel sick when I walk through A and E. At least staff move through it so quickly the current set of juniors don't recognize me as the troublemaker. The consultants do. But a few have told me that they are pleased I did it.'

'Weren't they embarrassed?'

'No, I don't think so. They thought the same as me. When someone actually does it...does something positive, everyone suddenly says "Yeah, I agree, it's unacceptable..." Like the emperor's new clothes, everyone pretends it's fine, they can manage, then someone pipes up and the truth becomes clear to all, undeniable. Weird psychology.'

'But why did it take your call? The Trust knew about the situation, the department was aware... not just from your comments... but it took the fear of a GMC investigation to do anything.'

'I honestly don't know.'

'Has anyone from senior management spoken to you?'

'Yep.'

'And...?'

'It was all very reasonable, understanding, respectful, in fact.'

'Fake?'

'Actually, no. We got into a good discussion. He made me feel relaxed, and we went into it in some detail.'

'Such as?'

'The bigger picture. He allowed me to push him... to draw him out... to reveal HIS thoughts about whistleblowing. It wasn't the greatest example of whistle-blowing in history was it, really – more of an alert I think – so I don't think he minded talking about it. So we got into the bigger picture. He encouraged me to think about scale, to think about the hospital as a unit, providing care to all its patients and to the whole community. Elective and emergency. Babies, kids... not just the sort of patient *I* was seeing. Those in charge have to decide where to put the resources, where to place the staff...'

'So only *they* have the overview, and the knowledge...'

'Perhaps, but it went further. I said yeah, you have to make hard decisions, to ration basically, but you in turn are being rationed, by the government, who have demanded that you save x million this year as a share of the £20 billion of efficiency savings. He liked that.'

'He didn't really agree to pass the buck onto the government, did he?'

'Not as such. But perhaps he should have. I might have sympathised with him.'

'You can take the bigger picture further, you know, Adam.'

'How?'

'To society as a whole. Why does the government demand we save £20 billion?'

'Because the economy is screwed. Austerity.'

'Yes, that's the environment we live in. But within that environment, the government has decided to squeeze the health service because it has a duty to maintain other parts of the state at the same time. Defense, social security, prisons... so in their eyes, the bigger picture demands that Trusts feel the pain. That's the price of austerity, of long-term economic stability. We don't have that overview, the *really* big overview.'

'You really believe that? No wonder *you* didn't make that call. You've intellectualised it to death.'

'Perhaps.'

'I said I sympathized with the big picture, but ultimately it doesn't cut it. Because it's not *our* business to care about the bigger picture, don't you see? Resources are to be sent down according to the best judgements or intentions of our political masters, or moved around the Trust by our senior managers, but we must concern ourselves with what the effect of those decisions is at ground level.'

'Humour me a minute, Adam; I'm not criticising you... but *why* whinge about those decisions? We *live* in the big picture. We are citizens in a democracy; we, as a society, voted for austerity and hardship. We ARE cogs. That's the state we're in; we should just do our best within it.'

'It doesn't matter. We, as doctors, work in a *small* world, the hospital... and we are there to make patients better. *We* are the ones with the eyes and the ears to tell the ones who move those resources around that their decisions are proving destructive. *We* are the ones who must tell them if minimum acceptable standards are not being maintained. Who else is going to spot that? If not us, who?'

'But doesn't everyone think that their little domain is under-resourced, straining to maintain minimum standards? We can't have all of them ringing the GMC helpline.'

'I agree. And that's why it took me a year. I challenged myself repeatedly, told myself it was just me, just a bad run of shifts, that my seniors had re-cognised the problem and were dealing with it... but nothing happened! So I did it. I reassured myself that it was up to me to tell them that here, in this case, the balance wasn't right.'

'Eyes and ears.'

'Yep. That's what Francis said.'

'And mouths too.'

It is deeply ironic that Robert Francis QC published his report *Freedom to speak up: an independent review on creating an open and honest reporting culture in the NHS* in February 2015, the same month that Chris Day entered his first employment tribunal and heard that there was no case for HEE to answer as he was not their employee. While Francis presented his report, which includes the sentence,

> That raising concerns is a positive, not a troublesome activity, and a shared commitment to support and encourage all those who raise honestly held concerns about safety

Dr Day was sent away without any hope of redress. The final irony is that QEH intensive care unit underwent peer review in February 2017 and was found to be deficient in its staffing.

> The Critical Care Unit at QEH had 8 beds when it opened in 2001. As a result of the mergers, and associated increased workload, it has expanded into adjacent ward areas and now runs 18 beds and an additional 19th bed as part of an escalation area. The unit has grown from 8 beds in 2001, to the 19 it has today, without any significant increase in resources over the time period.

> The perception on the unit was that there had been a significant in-crease in activity in recent years and subsequent increase in workload for medical team. This was felt to be a serious issue by review team as there did not appear to be a plan to address the consultant shortfall.

Chris Day was right all along.

iii. 'I'm not happy with this!' said the nurse in ED. She raised her voice above the undying tumult of pain and anxiety that fills departments between 6PM and midnight. My registrar, a surgeon, was trying to insert a chest drain, the same kind that I used on the ICU four years later. I was his junior. The patient, Simon, had a pneumothorax. His lungs were fragile and over-expanded be-cause of chronic, severe asthma. He had suffered a further asthma attack that evening, but instead of getting better with inhalers, it got much worse. His mother found him gasping for breath and in severe pain, clutching his right side. An ambulance rushed him in under a blue-light and deposited him in the resuscitation bay. Dave, my registrar, was called as soon as the chest x-ray confirmed that the right lung had burst, causing air to leak between the pleural membranes (just as blood was to accumulate in Maghadi Padam's case). As the pressure of the air rose, it squashed the lung and inhibited the usual expansion and deflation. The left lung was also being affected, as was his heart. All the structures in the chest were suffering. His blood pressure was falling; his lips were blue. Yet he was still conscious, and there was pure fear in his wide-open eyes.

Dave cut down between two ribs. Whatever the volume of local anaesthetic he had injected into the skin and tissues before pressing his scalpel, it was not enough. Simon was screaming. As his air and oxygen reserves dwindled, so did the volume. Soon, all he could do was whimper.

Dave was having trouble. As the surgeon on call, he was expected to know how to do this. (Later, I learned that ED staff and medical trainees should be able to do it too, hence my eagerness to master the skill; the technique has developed, and we would not use such a thick tube for this indication now.) It was taking too long. A swift, aggressive jab with the scalpel should have opened a way through the tissues. I could hear him muttering 'Black skin, it's tough sometimes.' I didn't know what to say to that, though I have since found that, indeed, black skin can be tougher to cut. I noticed the nurse at Simon's side. Her hands rested on his shoulders and her mouth was close to his ear, where she murmured comfort. But her words had no therapeutic effect. She straightened up, faced Dave, and said confidently,

'I'm not happy with this!'

It had taken courage for her to say anything. She was young, not one of the senior staff who had seen generations of trainees pass through the department. I could tell that every available moral fibre was employed in holding her spine and fixing her gaze at the surgical registrar. He paused, looked back at her, the rigid, shaking form of Simon between them, and said,

'Shut up! If I don't get this tube in, he's going to...' A residuum of delicacy stopped him from saying 'dead' over the patient.

'But he's in too much pain,' she countered.

'No... *time*!'

I didn't want to be there anymore. The atmosphere was sub-zero. Please God, I thought, let that tube go in.

The trocar passed through a fibrous layer and entered the pleural space. There was an audible rush of air as it escaped under pressure. The effect on Simon's oxygen levels was instantaneous. His pain subsided. His colour changed. He looked up at his surgeon with confusion. I hoped that the brief exchange of opinions had gone unheard.

Now that the emergency had passed, everybody could go about their usual business. I wrote the case up in Simon's notes, Dave wiped himself down, then moved on to the next patient (a lady with abdominal pain, well within his comfort zone) and the young nurse continued to attend to her patient.

Half an hour later, Dave and I walked out of the ED (an aged prefab unit, part of a hospital that had barely changed since the Second World War) and across the grass to the doctors' mess.

'That was tense,' I said.

'What?' (What!? Had the nurse's interjection made no impact on him?)

'Simon, his nurse. When she told you to stop.'

'Oh that. Very silly. Totally inappropriate.'

'But did you... did you use local?'

'Anaesthetic? No. There was no time. He could have arrested any second. He'll be fine.'

'Did you speak to her, the nurse?' In the deepening dusk, I looked across at him. The shape of his lips, the quizzical set of his profile, revealed that the thought had never crossed his mind.

'No. Why?'

I left it there. It was not my place to suggest a debrief, or to put the other side of the argument, that Simon's suffering had been so extreme it was quite possible that he would be forever damaged by the experience. And after all, hadn't the chest drain insertion taken so long, there had clearly been ample time for local anaesthetic to be given in the first place?

I left it there, made Dave a cup of coffee, and contemplated the list of patients I had to review before making an attempt to lie on the sofa.

One thing was clear to me, though: that nurse would never question a doctor again.

4.6 Tunnel

Remember my reaction to Charlie's error with the insulin?

> Isn't it obvious – I mean, for God's sake, Charlie, how did you think Mr Grey had been getting insulin up to this point?

For *God's* sake...

I am frequently presented with narratives of patient safety incidents. Often, my first reaction is 'Why, *why* did they do that?' For a long time, I found myself having to work through this phase until, by elevating myself above the incident, I was able to look down and see the bigger picture. Later, I discovered a book by Sidney Dekker, an Australian safety expert. There are many safety experts out there, but he writes in a lively and accessible way. There is little formal safety training in the NHS, so each of us must find what works best. The book was *The Field Guide to Human Error Investigations* (Ashgate, 2006). The chapter 'Reactions to failure: why the surprising nature of failure makes you revert easily to the bad apple theory' taught me that my blaming instinct was part of the typical 'old view' of human error that regards in-dividual behaviour as the main driver and as something to control. To control that slippery, unpredictable factor within an organisation you 'shape [] attitudes with posters and campaigns and sanctions...' There may even be 'bad apples' who always let the side down. The new view (not so new now – this philosophy is widely ac-cepted in the NHS) suggests that human error is a consequence of systems, a product of the organisation. As such, instances of failure are a source of information; they provide valuable insights into fallibilities that lie beneath, and such information is to be welcomed. Hence, we encourage incident reporting, DATIXs etc. We accept that healthcare staff 'do not come to work to do a bad job' and that 'as far as the people were concerned, the [bad] outcome was not going to happen. If they knew it was going to, they would have done something else' (the 'local rationality principle').

A true story told in the present tense: a trainee discharges a 72-year-old female patient from the ED with reassurance after she presented with abdominal pain and fever. At triage, there was no fever (in fact, her temperature was slightly low at 36.1°C; she had been sat outside in a draughty waiting room), but the first blood pressure was on the low side at 97 mmHg systolic and respiratory rate was raised to 25 breaths per minute. The doctor takes a thorough history, diagnoses a gastro-intestinal upset with mild dehydration and sends off bloods. The results are un-remarkable. The white cell count is normal. Blood pressure rises to 115 mmHg systolic after half a litre of intravenous saline. There is no fever on a second mea-surement. The patient feels better. There is no suspicion or physical evidence of sepsis, so the usual protocol or 'bundle' does not need to be instituted. The lady is sent home.

She comes back 6 hours later in a terrible state. She has been found on the floor unresponsive, clammy, with a very low blood pressure. Another doctor looks on the results system and finds that the CRP, a sensitive blood marker of infection, was hugely elevated at 360 mg/L. It was tested 6 hours ago. The previous doctor missed it! The patient goes to ICU for three weeks and makes a slow recovery from emergency surgery. She had an abdominal abscess caused by diverticular disease. It transpires that the CRP result was not on the system when the patient was discharged. The first doctor was confident that there was no serious underlying illness, based on examination and blood count. She didn't think there was anything seriously wrong. She didn't look it up later.

Here are some of my initial reactions to this 'failure':

- Why send off a blood test if you're not going to look at it? *Come on*, that's basic.
- If you're not going to wait for result to come back before you discharge, at least make a note and go back to check later. *Details, details.*
- In fact, looking at the notes, the patient's temperature (abnormally low), blood pressure and respiratory rate at admission were consistent with SIRS (systemic inflammatory response syndrome) – sepsis should have been suspected more strongly. This was a miss. The signs were there! *Sepsis is a killer!* Haven't you seen the media lately?
- Are this doctor's clinical antennae quite right? – she said the patient was 'normal' on examination, but come on, there must have been some tenderness or a mass. This will need to be forwarded to her educational supervisor. *Some doctors just don't recognise ill patients; maybe you're one of them.*

The focus of accountability and yes, blame, appears clear.

Dekker's scheme helps us look at this differently. Being a trained pilot and having been involved in investigations, he provides many aeronautical examples, but here I'll stick to the medical scenario.

He states that my initial reactions are bound to be:

- Retrospective – yes, guilty, how could it be otherwise?

- Counterfactual – I immediately focus on what 'could or should have done', rather than what actually happened, i.e., the actual facts; yes, guilty.
- Judgmental – guilty: I'm human, we all do it.
- Proximal – he means I am focused on the acts of the person closest to the patient and the incident. Yes, but where else would I start?

Now, with an effort, I delve into these tendencies.

Retrospection aka hindsight. Of course, the investigator will be looking at things backwards, but being aware of risks in this approach is the key. To me, it is obvious that a CRP of over 300 suggests sepsis; how could it not have been assimilated into the clinical decision? But Dekker describes how hindsight oversimplifies and makes events linear. Knowing the outcome, I can immediately see that failure to look up the CRP led to delayed diagnosis of the abscess. I am biased by knowing the outcome. In reality, the CRP was one of many, maybe hundreds, of pieces of information that the doctor was trying to assimilate during that shift in ED. The observer strips all the extraneous factors away to look at the critical steps related to the one patient, while the doctor was existing within a blur of activity and information. To put it simply, she was busy! But haven't we all been busy? Again, my response is judgmental.

Next – the *counterfactual*. 'They shouldn't have let the patient go without checking the CRP'. Why didn't those initial observations trigger a hunt for sepsis, in case she had SIRS (which causes fever and other sepsis signs but without underlying infection)? Look at the Trust guidance. If my role here is to work out why the patient went home without the correct diagnosis, Dekker asks, 'Why waste time on laying out what did not happen? The point in understanding human error is to find out why things happened the way they did.' This reminds me that the constructive approach is to explain what actually happened, rather than dwell on parallel universes where the 'right' thing happened. It's a subtle point, but useful. 'What people did... must have made sense to them given their goals, knowledge and attention at the time. Otherwise, like you, they would have done something else.'

But what about my accusation that a strong guideline (for sepsis) was overlooked? That's why we have guidelines, isn't it, to guide, to take away the variability of individual decision-making. Dekker would accuse me here of 'cherry-picking'. In any timeline leading to failure, it is possible to lift out certain facts that demonstrate non-compliance with an idealised approach. The same goes for 'standards of good practice' in general. When not met, we must immediately assume 'poor practice', because you have 'substituted your own [calm, controlled, clear] world for the one that surrounded the people in question.'

Judgmental – here we get to the nitty gritty. From my elevated position, I see the patient lying on the trolley in the ED, the abscess growing inside them just waiting to release its pus into the abdomen, I watch the blood taken and sent to the lab, I see the doctor reassure the lady that there isn't much to worry about, I see the CRP result arrive on the system, just begging to be read... but the doctor is off seeing other patients now... it's so frustrating. I am emotionally involved.

Again, my role should be to understand how it happened. The means standing in the doctor's shoes. I need to know what it feels like to run around that department, multi-tasking, reprioritising constantly, assimilating signals. Signals which may have been obscured, like the 'infamous' signal 109 at Ladbroke Grove[43] which could easily be missed among the clutter of overhead lines and other signs. Perhaps this CRP was like that. It didn't ping, it didn't flash, it just sat among all the normal results failing to attract attention to itself.

Dekker's final subheading is *'Proximal'*, which refers to our tendency to focus immediately on the actions of the person who was present and who seems to have 'caused' the incident. The difference between the 'sharp' and 'blunt' ends of an organisation is simple enough to understand. The blunt end is the system, the part of an organisation that created the circumstances in which the doctor failed. In the NHS, we are used to taking this broader view. Our root cause analysis methodologies, such as '5-Whys' and 'Fishbone', encourage us to ask deeper questions. We get there in the end. But still, it takes some discipline to pull back from the more emotional 'Why, oh why?' stage.

In this example, having obtained the doctor's own account, I might ask:

- Why was the patient discharged without a diagnosis? – would a system of mandatory consultant review help?
- Why was nobody alerted to the abnormal CRP result? – should there be a policy of the lab phoning through grossly abnormal values?
- Why wasn't the patient informed that some results were pending? – should the discharge letter make it clear that some results are awaited?
- Was the doctor over-burdened with cases? How many did she see that night? Is there a staffing issue in the ED?
- Was there pressure to discharge?

The last two are recurring themes in the NHS. Later in his book, Dekker describes NASA's seemingly unachievable mantra 'faster, better and cheaper': hitting more than two out of three seems impossible. In a busy ED, we want faster turnarounds, high diagnostic accuracy, good clinical outcomes, but fewer scans and tests, if possible, please! As an investigator, I know that finishing off a report with the observation that more staff are required will be to add a drop into the national ocean of resource demand. More ingenious solutions are required.

Why write this when Dekker's argument is already won? Well, the argument may not be won. The balance between personal accountability and ultimate responsibility of the 'system' has not yet been found. I have explored blame and accountability and have found that the answers are not always easy to find. The case of Hadiza Bawa Garba is the most prominent example. It is not so easy to take the broad, non-individual view from the outset. Those working in patient safety know, despite the work of Dekker and others, that individual variation exists. If a system works well most of the time, should that system be changed at great expense and upheaval after a failure, or the individual? This train of thought brings us to just culture, restorative justice and forward-looking accountability.

4.7 Rainstorm

A response to seeing doctors go to prison.

He parked his car and turned off the radio. '... *doctors will be criminalised if found guilty of willful negligence...*' — was the sentence echoing in his mind as he entered the hospital through a side door. He was on-call today, but he hoped to see some of his own patients before things began to heat up. His first patient had been diagnosed with inoperable lung cancer, and their relatives were on the ward waiting to talk to him. David took them into a private room. As he closed the door behind them the patient's daughter pre-empted him, asking,

'Who are you?'

'I'm David Clark, the SHO.'

She opened a spiral bound notebook and began to take notes.

'... before you go on, doctor, can you tell me when you found the lump?'

'Well... soon after he came in, when he had the scan...'

'Wasn't it on the x-ray he had on the day he came to casualty?'

'Well, yes, but we – the doctors looking after him them – were concentrating on the infection, but now a scan has proved it is...'

'That was two weeks ago. I don't understand why there has been a delay.'

David controlled himself. His plan – the careful steps he rehearsed in order to take the family along an explanatory path of diagnosis, treatment options, arrangements, support – had been blown to bits. Flustered, he continued. Everything was being written down. A phrase from the cop shows rattled in his head as he tried to focus on the words, '...*will be used against you in a court of law...*'

The day got busier. While he was inserting a urinary catheter he was fast-bleeped to another ward. He couldn't move, committed to the task that he had begun. He hurried it, didn't do it quite as carefully as he normally would, anxious to leave the patient and rush to the emergency. When he got to the other ward a charge nurse informed him that he had no choice but to fill an incident form. Only the most junior member of the team had responded to the urgent call, and she hadn't been able to deal with the emergency.

'But I was tied up; I couldn't come...'

'I know, doctor. But we have to do these forms. Otherwise nothing changes, does it...?'

He imagined his name in the text, the focus of culpability. In the Acute Medical Unit ward, he received a call; the bed manager had been trying to find him. There was a patient on an outlying ward under his team's care who had not been reviewed for four days. Although David was mired in emergency admissions by now (enjoying the rapid throughput of fresh cases, stimulated by the need to make fast decisions, arrange investigations and take responsibility for the treatment plans), he dragged himself away to visit the lost patient. She was very elderly, evidently succumbing to pneumonia on a background of heart disease. In fact, the admitting team had done a very thorough job. They had spoken to the family, discussed resuscitation, introduced the idea of palliative care, but then...nothing. For *four* days. No doctors. The odd on-call visit to prescribe fluids, but nothing substantive. It shouldn't happen, but it can and it does. And now her son was here, visibly upset. David introduced himself. The son retorted,

'I want an explanation!'

'I'm sorry, there must have been a mix up, and then over the weekend...'

'I don't care. No-one has seen her; she's been ignored. Who is this?' He pointed to the consultant's name written in a blue marker on the white sign above the bed, 'Is he the consultant?'

'She. Yes, she is. But your mother has only just come under her care.'

'No, she hasn't; that name has been up there every day. But you didn't see her on Monday or Tuesday. It's neglect. What chance she did have has been lost.'

'The nurses tell me she has been comfortable.'

'Yes, she has. But...

David entered the final hours of his difficult day. He made many accurate diagnoses and many good decisions. The consultant seemed happy with his clerking, but David was down. He kept thinking back to the old lady's son, his sharp words. 'Willful...' 'Ignored...' 'Neglected...' David's usual spark had been extinguished. His shift was over. As he walked into the doctors' room to pick up his coat the bleep went off one last time. He called the number.

'Dr Clark. Hi, it's Mary on Chestnut ward. Mr Threlfall, the man we put out a fast bleep for earlier, he's died. No, it was expected, your registrar came to see him and made him not for resuscitation. It's just, because of that incident form earlier, I'm going to send the notes on to the morbidity and mortality meeting for review. As a formality, you know.'

As he closed the door of the office behind him a colleague ran past him in the corridor; breathlessly he shouted,

'Crash call. Some guy who had a catheter inserted this morning, on warfarin, he's bleeding out...'

David opened his car door, sat heavily in the seat, and turned on the radio. —*'Police have confirmed a second criminal investigation into a potentially avoidable death in Mid Staffordshire, five years after...'*— He turned it off, put his palms on the steering wheel and his forehead on the backs of his hands, and muttered, 'I can't do this anymore.'

David sat in his consultant's office. She had locked the door and asked that they not be disturbed. She had heard about his decision and started by asking him to hear her out. Then she explored what it was that had made up his mind. He described his shift from hell. She said,

'I'll tell you what I think. We've got to help you adapt to these... stresses. The scrutiny, the incident reporting...'

'You mean, just ignore it?'

'In a way, yes. They should not dictate how you function as a doctor. Because they are more visible – after Mid Staffs, after the Francis Report – and because they have imposed themselves on you, you have come to react to *them* rather than the instincts that drew you into this vocation in the first place. They are important, yes; they are there to protect patients, yes – but from those doctors who might be harmful. You are not one of those doctors. You are good. You should be able to function without being fearful of running into these electric fences and getting hurt all the time. From what I've seen of the way you practise medicine, you'll find a path that does not veer too close to the edge of reasonable, sensible practice.'

'Yet I seem to have run into those fences time and again. I described it to my girlfriend as living in a continuous rainstorm, where each raindrop is a new patient and a potential clinical incident or mistake that I must protect myself from. Usually I can, using my knowledge and experience, or luck, but sometimes one of those raindrops gets through, and explodes. And I never know which one it's going to be...'

'What happens to patients isn't always down to you or your decisions. Some get sick despite everything. You can't necessarily stop that, so you can't take the blame. Looking back, did you actually do anything *wrong* during that entire on call?'

'I felt like I did. Incident forms, threats of 'willful negligence'! And the catheter. That was my fault.'

'Didn't you hear? He had a bladder tumour, that's why he bled! Forget that. And 'wilful negligence'... please don't be scared by that term. The relative who used it wasn't criticising you; he didn't know who you were. He was frustrated with the situation. Wouldn't you be? That term, whatever it means, wasn't designed to be applied to isolated mistakes.'

'But she *was* neglected.'

'Yes, by our system – and we've tried to close that gap. But not by you. You were never in danger. Did you really think you could go to jail? Really?'

'No. Yes. I don't know. I just kept hearing it...'

'I know. And the incident form... well, they are important, and are used to alert us – the doctors who will be working here for years! – about what needs to be fixed. That wasn't personal either.'

'I appreciate what you're saying, I really do. But I can't work in this atmosphere of... negativity.'

'But it's just that. An atmosphere. We have to learn to breathe it without taking it personally, without a sense of suffocation.'

'So, it's my fault – this crisis. I've got it out of perspective?'

'A bit. That's why we're talking. I want to help you understand how a good doctor must accept that they *will* be subject to what seems like criticism now and again. You seem to be aware of your limitations. In fact, you may be *too* aware, because you've grown nervous of them. The warnings and safety nets that have become so much more visible recently are not there to punish you. If you, as one of the great majority of trainee doctors who are good, intelligent and conscientious, are picked out and quoted in some incident form, or referred to anonymously in a mortality meeting, it's more likely to be a reflection of how stressed the service is, or how fallible a particular system is. It's not a judgement on *you*.'

'But if I am a good doctor, why am I being reminded about these systems all the time –threatened by them?'

'There is a temptation to use them as levers, to get you to see patients more urgently than you, as the doctor, might feel is appropriate. Remember, you are the doctor; your opinion is valuable. If you are asked to see someone who is deteriorating, you have the right, by virtue of your experience and understanding of clinical priorities, to decide how soon they should be seen. But if somebody else thinks they should be seen sooner, and they are able to wield a stick, it's natural for them to do this to motivate you to hurry up. They want their patient seen first – that's natural. But in doing so, they ensure that you are driven by a negative motivation rather a positive one. You fear the situation rather than embrace it. And look where it has brought you.'

'So, I just say no, sorry; I'll come when I want to?'

'If you are juggling what appear to be equally important priorities, yes. But you must explain why – help the person you are talking to understand and, if possible, agree. And you must follow through, see that patient, hold your course, finish each task that you begin, and leave the ward confident that you have dealt with the problem in hand...'

'And when I get called away to see an even sicker patient...'

'Ask, build a picture, make your own mind up. Things don't happen that fast. The sicker patient will have been deteriorating all night; they can usually wait another 10 minutes. If they are arresting you will find out; there will be a crash call. It's all about accommodating the continuous stream of emergencies, catching the raindrops, without being caught up and carried away in the flow. If you do, you will become disorientated. You are the one who needs to keep calm, maintain perspective. It's you they're looking to for reassurance. Remember that, David.'

'I hadn't thought about it like that. I've just felt... so junior... all the time.'

'Junior in some ways, but senior in so many others... at three in the morning you are the most accessible doctor on the wards. First contact. It's a massive responsibility. With that responsibility comes respect.'

'Really? I don't feel it.'

'It comes.'

'If there was respect, they wouldn't have done an incident form.'

'No. You're taking it the wrong way – personally. The incident form is irrelevant. It wasn't a judgement on you; it was an observation that when a fast bleep was put out the doctor couldn't come because he was doing something else. So what? If you can accept that now and again, purely by virtue of the fact that you see so many patients, you are *bound* to be involved in a complaint or an incident form, you will be able to work naturally, learn and progress. If you can accept that you work within a network of continuous feedback, but without having your outlook obscured by it, you will achieve whatever you want to achieve.'

'You make it sound almost cosy. It isn't. In the middle of the night I get shouted at if I don't come. And relatives write down what I'm saying as though everything is a statement.'

'Well... so might you when you have a relative in hospital. Are you coming back to work next week?'

'I haven't decided.'

'That's OK; take your time.'

Summing Up

How can a doctor thrive in an atmosphere so heavy with risk? As I tried to emphasise at the beginning of this book, positive experiences will usually outweigh the negative, but only the wounds leave scars. The good times sustain you through the hard times and remind you why you wanted to be a doctor. This is easy for me to say. I am nearly 50. I rarely feel endangered or vulnerable. I think – though there is still time for me to be proven wrong – that a conscientious approach, experience and seniority will insulate me from accusations of negligence even if I do make mistakes in the future. So, as I lean back from the keyboard, this catalogue of error nearly done, the dangers of being a doctor appear diminished. But what of those who are just starting their careers? Do I really understand what they are going through on the wards? For there is another danger – that of experienced (dare I say, battle-hardened?) veterans underestimating the impact of errors on those more junior to them. In an old fashioned way, I might find myself thinking – *if I got through it without falling apart, you can too*. Might? No. I *do*, already. Just the other day I was discussing a serious incident that involved a trainee. We were planning the investigation. The potential damage that interviews or requests for 'an account of events' would do to young doctors and nurses was raised by a colleague. I said, 'That's something they will need to learn to deal with. They will be involved in many investigations during their careers. We'll support them, obviously. It's not pleasant... but it's necessary.'

Phrases like 'snowflake' are used to describe doctors who just can't take the heat. Pejorative references are made about millennials and Generation Z; next, I understand, is Gen α. Resilience, as we have seen, is a dirty word. The onus is not on doctors to cope, but on the system to support them. Maybe I *am* too old now to fully understand. Perhaps, because I never reached a crisis point (persistent thoughts of resignation, alternative careers, or worse), I am not qualified to comment. I have never cried at work, but that probably doesn't mean anything. I do find myself thinking – yeah, I've been there. You'll be okay. I'm here to support you, I do believe you are a good doctor with a great future, but resilience is a genuine attribute and it derives from an internal source of energy, deep in your moral core, one that you must learn to access on your own, during the dark hours when you contemplate the consequences of your errors or omissions.

Not a very helpful attitude, perhaps. There must be something more I can do. A fundamental lesson, a surefire strategy, a psychological gambit, something that I can hand on.

What is it?

It is this: error is inevitable; you *will* make mistakes. The mistakes that you make, and the pain that they cause you, are part of the deal you made in choosing a high stakes profession. The mistakes you make will not spoil deals, wipe shares, spill oil, undersell land, obscure justice, ruin experiments or crash cars... but they will diminish others' wellbeing and sometimes shorten their lives. Although some of the

DOI: 10.1201/9781003189824-101

mistakes may have a root cause in a hitherto unrecognised deficiency in the system, others will be the result of personal misjudgements, erroneous assumptions, disorganisation or knowledge gaps. There may be an explanation that has nothing whatsoever to do with you, but you will not be able to dissociate yourself from blame entirely. Therefore, the wounds and the scars that you suffer *should* be felt; you *have* to notice them. However, in order for you to remain mentally healthy (and useful to other patients), those scars cannot be allowed to impair or paralyse you. Your mind needs to move freely, and the next patient in line cannot see the fibrous reaction. To achieve this, your seniors, the medical establishment and society must help. You are owed something, for without your willingness to practice in this high-stakes world, society's diseases will go untreated. You have a right to assistance in healing and learning. You deserve the benefit of the doubt and a commitment not to rush to blame.

As shown in the chapters on David Sellu and Hadiza Bawa Garba, society is not there yet. Its fossilised ways have trouble keeping up with real life on the wards, where computers often do not work, results are delayed or messages lost, where technologies from the 1970s (like bleeps) are still relied upon, where the gap between ideal and real staffing levels remains laughable and archaic cultures do not provide the oversight that you need and deserve. Working in public service means working in a constrained environment. But in most hospitals, I believe, there is a genuine desire to support you. The people around you will have experienced similarly sleepless nights and intrusive thoughts. There is understanding.

The saving strategy, I believe, is to face your errors, reflect (with help, if needed) and regard each scar as a badge. Proof that you were there. Proof that you learned. For each psychological adjustment, each procedural trick, each newly recognised pattern of symptoms, signs and data, each anecdote, each memory, will count as an accomplishment towards the ultimate goals: expertise, wisdom, and the ability to teach the generation that follows.

Endnotes

1. The 'Citadel' is the medical establishment, which Andrew eventually conquers through hard work and a direct, uncompromising medical manner. To gain entry he must pass become a Member of the Royal College of Physicians, by passing the MRCP exam. At the *viva voce* or oral exam, Andrew is asked what fundamental principle he has borne in mind during his career. He answers, '... never to take anything for granted'. Emma, the fictional doctor who failed to check a microbiology result in introduction to this book, learned the same principle the hard way. In *The Citadel* Cronin describes a 'free at the point of service' local health scheme, based on subscriptions. This model inspired aneurin Bevan to create the National Health Service (NHS).
2. 'When you hear hoofbeats behind you, don't expect to see a zebra', attributed to Theodore E. Woodward (1914–2005), American physician and researcher. He meant, beware of making exotic or rare diagnoses when another, more commonplace disease is statistically far more likely.
3. The four-hour target was introduced by a Labour government in 2004 and was intended to keep patients flowing through Emergency Departments (ED), thus reducing the unacceptably long waiting times. It was largely effective but put clinicians and managers under great pressure. ED doctors resisted moves by the Conservative government in 2020 to scrap it.
4. Peritonitis is infection within the abdominal lining. It is generally lethal without surgical intervention.
5. DNACPR – Do Not Attempt Cardiopulmonary Resuscitation, otherwise known as DNR, NFR or even AND (Allow Natural Death). AND is increasingly favoured, as it emphasises a positive approach, allowing nature to do what it must inevitably do at some point without medical staff getting in the way and inflicting more discomfort, rather than depriving patients of a treatment.
6. Asystole means a complete absence of cardiac activity.
7. TURP – transurethral resection of the prostate. A metal pipe containing a camera is inserted into the penis up to the prostate, allowing the enlarged lobe to be scraped away.
8. 'query aspiration' – aspiration pneumonia means that the lung infection has been caused by food or drink going into the trachea or windpipe rather than the oesphagus; this happens when the muscles that control swallowing do not work properly.

9. 'schisto' – schistosomiasis, a parasitic flatworm acquired in water contaminated by freshwater snails. Africa sees the greatest number of deaths. The worms can move to the liver and lead to symptoms similar to cirrhosis, especially the build-up of fluid, or ascites, in the abdomen.

10. Gawande was a lead investigator in a large, international trial that measured surgical complications before and after a 19-item checklist was introduced. Overall post-operative death rate fell from 1.5 to 0.8%. This equates to 1.6 million lives saved annually if, as the authors suggest in the *New England Journal of Medicine* paper (*NEJM* 2009; 360:491–499), 234 million operations are performed worldwide each year.

11. The term 'turf', meaning the transfer of responsibility of a patient to an alternative doctor or team, became common after the publication of *The House of God* by Samuel Shem (Richard Marek Publishers, 1978), that famous account of dehumanisation in medicine. It is not clear whether Shem invented the term, or just reproduced it. Probably the latter.

12. I am very critical of this book (Picador, 2017). In fact, I despise its unprofessional attacks on perceived patient characteristics such as obesity, (lack of) intelligence or religious belief. He would, I am sure, have been struck off if he had not already removed himself from the medical register. However, in common with the tens of thousands who have read it, I was also moved. And of course, I read it right to the end. It is an important book.

13. David Hare's play *Stuff Happens* (2004) examines the arguments for and against the invasion of Iraq in 2003.

14. Scott SD, Hirschinger LE, Cox KR, et al., The natural history of recovery for the healthcare provider "second victim" after adverse patient events, *BMJ Quality & Safety* 2009;18:325–330.

15. Sir Robert Francis led the inquiry into another major NHS scandal. Due to the tireless work of Julie Bailey, whose mother died in Mid-Staffordshire NHS Foundation Trust, dangerously poor quality of care was revealed. Francis highlighted issues with a target-based management culture and the failure of medical and nursing staff to act when they observed unacceptable standards (*Report of the Mid Staffordshire NHS Foundation Trust Public Inquiry*, 2013).

16. Berwick D, *A promise to learn – a commitment to act: improving the safety of patients in England.* London, 2013: Department of Health.

17. The NHS grades harm as follows:
    Low: Any unexpected or unintended incident that required extra observation or minor treatment and caused minimal harm to one or more persons receiving NHS-funded care. *Moderate*: Any unexpected or unintended incident that resulted in a moderate increase in treatment, possible surgical intervention, cancelling of treatment, or transfer to another area, and which caused significant but not permanent harm, to one or more persons receiving NHS-funded care. *Severe*: Any unexpected or unintended incident that appears to have resulted in permanent harm to one or more persons.

18. Zander Swinburbe, *The Independent* newspaper, 9.3.2014.

19. In May 2017 Ian Paterson was imprisoned for wilfully wounding seventeen women through 'botched and unnecessary' breast operations. He is thought to have harmed hundreds more. Kennedy's report into his practice found that concerns had been raised in 2003, but that no action was taken by his employers (Professor Sir Ian Kennedy, Review of the Response of Heart of England NHS Foundation Trust to

Concerns about Mr Ian Paterson's Surgical Practice; Lessons to be Learned; and Recommendations).

20. Wilson JA, Unsupervised surgical training: questionnaire study, *BMJ* 1997; 314:1803.
21. Jagsi R, Lehmann LS, The ethics of medical education *BMJ* 2004; 329: 332.
22. Le Morvan P, Stock B, Medical learning curves and the Kantian ideal. *J Med Ethics* 2005 Sep;31(9):513–518.
23. CEA – a financial bonus awarded to NHS consultants who can demonstrate that they are working 'above and beyond' their contracted duties.
24. *What Doctors Feel: How Emotions Affect the Practice of Medicine* (Beacon Press, 2013).
25. Henry Bodkin, 'Doctors living in fear of fatal mistakes due to NHS pressures', says BMA, The *Daily Telegraph* 25.6.2018.
26. Cohen D, Back to blame: the Bawa-Garba case and the patient safety agenda, *BMJ* 2017; 359.
27. Gerarda C. et al., Making doctors better, *BMJ* editorial, 3.10.2018.
28. Reason J, Human error: models and management, *BMJ* 2000, Mar18; 320(7237):768–770.
29. For Doctors, Delving Deeper as a Way to Avoid Burnout, *The New York Times*, 10.10.2018.
30. Peters D, Horn C, Gishen F, Ensuring our future doctors are resilient, *BMJ* 2018; 362:2877.
31. Gerada edited the book *Beneath the White Coat: Doctors, Their Minds and Mental Health* (CRC Press, 2020) which explores the effects of witnessing suffering, involvement in safety incidents and citation in formal complaints on doctors' wellbeing.
32. Balme E, Gerada C, Page L, Doctors need to be supported, not trained in resilience, *BMJ* 2015; 351:h4709.
33. The problems of being a millennial doctor, *Pulse*, 22.2.2017.
34. Abandon the term "second victim", Clarkson MD, Haskell H, Hemmelgarn C et al., *BMJ* 2019; 364.
35. *The Sunday Times,* May 19, 2019.
36. Haemoptysis means coughing up blood from the lungs. Some cancers in the throat or neck can erode into major arteries, resulting in sudden, high volume, fatal haemoptysis. I will never forget comforting a junior colleague who observed a patient die from this complication during her first year as doctors on the ward. All she could do was place dark coloured blankets on his bed so that the gouts of crimson did not show up so much and add to his distress. The man faded over several minutes, falling into unconsciousness before dying. It was a blessed release. My colleague was 23 years old; she had been a doctor for three weeks.
37. All NHS employees (but not GPs) are protected by NHS indemnity: 'NHS bodies are liable at law for the negligent acts and omissions of their staff in the course of their NHS employment: Under NHS Indemnity, NHS bodies take direct responsibility for costs and damages arising from clinical negligence where they (as employers) are vicariously liable for the acts and omissions of their health care professional staff.' [From NHS Resolution, the body responsible for dealing with claims against the NHS.]
38. Previously mentioned in this book for his part in revealing the Bristol Heart scandal, many know Dr Hammond as a comedian. He has also campaigned on the treatment of whistle-blowers and misdiagnosis by pathologists.
39. Written reflection is dead in the water, *BMJ* 2016; 353:i3250.

40. Elective patients are those admitted by prior arrangement for planned surgery or procedures. They are inherently low risk, compared to patients admitted as emergencies.

41. The MPTS conducts tribunals into the professional standards of doctors who are referred to the GMC. It employs around 300 lay and professional members to make impartial decisions on whether doctors should be suspended. It is independent of the GMC, though this separation is relatively recent. In the case of Bawa-Gaba, the GMC and the MPTS came to legal blows, with the MPTS recommending suspension after the GNM verdict, while the GMC maintained that such a sentence should automatically lead to her being struck permanently off the register.

42. In this context 'resuscitation' means the administration of fluid to boost blood pressure and circulation, rather than restarting the heart with electricity.

43. The Ladbroke Grove (or Paddington) crash on October 5th 1999 caused 31 deaths and injured 417. Signal 109 had been 'passed at danger' on eight occasions over the previous six years, and the Cullen inquiry found that the low angle of the sun combined with poor sight lines led the driver to miss the red signal.

Index

abdominal pain, 51, 113, 125
accountability, 92–93, 96, 103, 104, 127
Acute Medical Unit, 43, 128
adrenaline, 4, 17, 19, 83, 84
ageing, 32
aggressive surgeon, 116
alcoholic cardiomyopathy, 10
alcoholism, 27, 34–35
Also Human: The Inner Lives of Doctors
      (2018), 95
anaemia, 23, 24
anaesthetic, 3, 6, 7, 17, 28, 54, 123, 124
AND (Allow Natural Death), 135n5
anecdotal memory, 13
anecdote, 13, 134
aneurysms, 39, 40, 80, 81
anger, 26, 40, 45, 75, 78, 89, 107
angry grief, 79
antibiotics, ix, 10, 18–20, 40–44, 73, 76, 90, 93,
      113, 114, 116
anti-coagulants, 27, 28
anti-parasitic agent, 12
aortic aneurysms, ruptured, 80, 81
apology, 40, 69, 70–76, 116
arrhythmia, 15
arterial blood, 2, 4, 51
arthritic hip bones, 3
arthritis, 3
asystole, 16, 17, 135n6
Atonement (2001), 84
attitude of patient, 75
avoidable error, 75

bacteria, ix, 18, 43
bad news, 31, 32, 34, 37, 48
Balme E, 137n32
*Beneath the White Coat: Doctors, Their Minds
      and Mental Health* (2020), 137n31
Berwick D, 67, 92, 136n16
bile duct, 48, 65–66, 70, 86, 88
      cutting, 53

infection in, 52
blame, 53, 91, 92, 93, 94, 96–98, 103–105, 109,
      111, 115, 134
bleeding ulcers, 83
blood clots, 87
blood lactate level, 108
blood pressure, 3–7, 26, 66, 76, 108, 113, 116,
      125, 138n42
blood thinners, 27, 28, 87, 88
blood vessel, ruptured, 63
Bodkin, Henry, 137n25
bone marrow cancer, 18
borderline decisions, 90
'botched and unnecessary' breast operations,
      136n19
bowel ischaemia, 52
brain, parasite in, 13
brain haemorrhage, 40
brain surgery, 64
Bringing Out The Dead (1999), x
Bristol Heart Babies Action Group, 82
Brown-Sequard syndrome, 2
burnout, 95, 99, 100

cancer, 9, 20–21, 65
      bone marrow, 18
      gastric, 20
      liver, 33
      lung, 128
      oesophageal, 53
      pancreatic, 47, 89
      rectal, 23
      stomach, 20
cancer cells, 33
cannula, 2, 3, 16, 25, 74, 117
cardiac arrest, 5, 37, 40, 52, 55, 73, 87, 106
cardiogenic shock, 67, 75
cardiothoracic surgery, 82, 85
central line insertions, 2, 74
cerebral haemorrhage, 39
checklist, 27–30, 136n10

chemotherapy, 47, 65
chest drain, 5, 6, 25, 54, 59, 74, 122, 124
chest infection, 36, 40, 41, 72, 84
chest pain, 74, 107
chlorhexidine, 6
cholangitis, 52
cholecystectomy, 53
Churg – Strauss syndrome, 12, 14
cirrhosis, 10, 23, 54, 113, 115
The Citadel (1937), 1, 135n1
Clarkson, Melissa, 99, 137n34
clinical fodder, 86
clotting, 5, 7, 8
Cohen D, 137n26
Collateral Damage (2010), 66
Collins, William, xii
colonoscopy, 23
coma, 5, 24, 25, 77, 88, 107
communication, failures in, 31
    comfort, 34–35
    cruel, 35–39
    dance, 47–49
    edge, 46–47
    limit, 31–32
    loose, 39–40
    low, 45–46
    privacy, 42–43
    proximity, 32–33
    radius, 33–34
    signals, 40–42
    unwanted, 43–45
*Complications: A Surgeon's Notes on an
        Imperfect Science* (2002), 86
'conduct' issues, 119
conscientious approach, 133
coronavirus, 23
counterfactual, 126
courage, 51, 101, 110, 123
Courvoisier's triad, 65
COVID-19 pandemic, xiv
Cox KR, 136n14
CPR, 17, 40, 45, 46
craniotomy, 81
Cronin AJ, 1, 135n1
Crown Prosecution Service, 113
CRP, 80, 125, 126, 127
crystalloid, 4
Cutting for Stone (2009), 34
cystic duct, cutting, 53

Dacre, Dame Jane Elizabeth, 1
DATIX, 1
Day, Chris, 119, 122
dead gut, 51, 52
dead legs, 80

Dean, Wendy, 98
death, 35, 46
dehydration, 125
Dekker, Sidney, 124, 125, 126, 127
de-stigmatisation, 101
detachment, 56
dextrose, 74
diabetic ketoacidosis, 77
diagnoses, correct, 1–2
diagnostic mistake, 75
'diffident' surgeon, 115–116
disappointment, 75, 94
distress, 19, 38, 46, 100, 101, 137n36
district general hospital (DGH), 79–81
diuretic, 4
DNACPR, 16, 37, 42, 45–46, 135n5
dobutamine, 4–5
Down's syndrome, 108
drinking, 34, 42, 63
*Drive: The Surprising Truth About What
        Motivates Us* (2009), 96
Dussek, Julian, 85
Duty of Candour, 67, 74–76

echocardiogram, 10, 17
eclampsia, 5
educational meeting, 80
educational supervisor, 68, 75, 93, 98, 103, 110
effective doctor, being, 52
elderly patients, ix, 3, 72
Elton, Caroline, 95
emergency department (ED), 62–64, 135n3
emergency surgery, 80
emotional pain, 33
empathy, 33, 43, 48, 65
Employment Rights Act, 119
enalapril, 108
endocarditis, 65
end-of-life type discussion, 41
endoscopy, 8, 9, 23, 35, 53, 62, 65, 83–84
eosinophils, 11, 12, 13
equanimity, 67
error, 75, 76, 97, 103, 111, 133
    and acceptable variation, 82
    avoidable, 75
    drug error, 68
    honest, 93
    human error, 124, 126
    individual, 79, 110
everyday stress, 99
expectation management, 79
experience, 96, 75, 81, 86, 95, 96, 133

feedback, 77, 90, 131
fever, 3–4, 11

The Field Guide to Human Error Investigations
 (2006), 124
florid crackles, 4
four-hour target, 135n3
Francis, Sir Robert, 67, 136n15
Frankl, Victor, 96

gallbladder, swollen, 65
gall bladder operation, 86
Garba, Hadiza Bawa, 91, 108, 109, 111,
 127, 134
gastric cancer, 20
Gawande, Atul, 29–30, 86, 136n10
General Medical Council (GMC), 82–83, 91, 96,
 103, 105, 107, 108, 110, 111, 112,
 120, 138n41
General Practitioner (GP), 25–26
'Generation Y' trainees, 98
gentamicin, 18, 19, 93
Gerada C, 96, 97, 137n31, 137n32
Gerarda C, 137n27
Gishen F, 96, 137n30
glycine, 18
Goddard, Andrew, 98
GREATIX, 1
grief, 34, 51, 53, 75, 78, 79, 89
Gross Negligence Manslaughter (GNM), 91,
 108, 115
guinea pigs, 86, 87

haemofiltration, 6–7, 19, 51, 66
haemoglobin level, 7
haemoptysis, 137n36
haemorrhage, cerebral, 39
haemorrhagic stroke, 31
hard news, delivering, 35
Hare, David, 136n13
Hartmann's procedure, 81
Haskell H, 137n34
headache, 3, 72
Health Education England (HEE), 119
heart attack, 10, 40, 53, 74, 94
heart damage, 4
heart surgery, 82
Hemmelgarn C, 137n34
hepatitis C virus, 54
hidden curriculum, 96
Hirschinger LE, 136n14
honest error, 93
Horn C, 96, 137n30
hospital at night, 59–62
hospitalisation, 26, 58, 72
The House of God (1978), 136n11
human error, 124, 126
hypoglycaemic coma, 77

ignorance, admitting, 15
immune systems of elderly patients, ix
individual errors, 79
infamy, on judgement and punishment, 103
 cross, 103–105
 Jack, 108–112
 maw, 112–116
 peer, 105–108
 rainstorm, 127–131
 tunnel, 124–127
 whistle, 116–124
infarcted, 4
infection
 bile duct, 52
 chest, 36, 40, 41, 72, 84
 kidney, 3
 urinary, ix, 11, 116
information gathering, 104
inkling, 32
inotropes, 21
insulin, 74, 76, 77, 97, 124
intensive care unit (ICU), ix, 4–6, 10

Jagsi R, 86, 137n21
jaundice, 24, 26, 34, 42, 48, 52, 62, 65
judgmental, 126

Kantian ideal, 87
Kay, Adam, 51, 99
Kennedy, Ian, 83, 85, 136n19
kidney failure, 18, 88–89
kidney infection, 3
known complication, 74, 104

Ladbroke Grove crash, 126, 138n43
LanguageLine, 37
learning, x, 1, 112
learning curve, 82, 84–86
Lehmann LS, 137n21
Le Morvan P, 87, 137n22
leukaemia, 6
liver, enlarged, 39
liver cancer, 33
liver disease, 23, 39
liver failure, 5, 14, 56
liver transplantation, 5, 34, 85
low blood pressure, 3–5, 10, 125
lumbar punctures (LP), 2–4, 61
lung, with fluid, 17
lung cancer, 128

Malek, Nishma, 98
Mannix, Kathryn, xiii
Marsh, Henry, 72
mask ventilation, 21

McEwan, Ian, 84
Medical Practitioners Tribunal Service (MPTS),
    113, 138n41
#medicineisgreat, 1
meeting
    educational, 80
    one-to-one, 107
meningococcal sepsis, 110
mesenteric ischaemia, 51
messenger, 48–49
misdiagnoses, 90
mistaken actions and reactions
    burn, 27–30
    flying, 1–2
    ignorant, 14–16
    listen, 8–10
    paralysis, 19–22
    patterns, 10–14
    pride, 5–8
    prison, 24–27
    shock, 3–5
    slick, 2–3
    stop, 16–17
    trust, 18–19
    wait, 17–18
    zone, 23–24
mistakes, x, xi, 103, 133
    avoiding making, 15
    diagnostic, 75
mitral valve, 67
modulating the degree of openness, 73
moral injury, 98–101
morphine, 33, 48, 88, 89
motivational approach, 3
Mukherjee, Siddhartha, 96

Nagpaul, Chaand, 91
naloxone, 89
National confidential Enquiry into Patient
        outcome and Death (NCEPOD), 46
National Health Service (NHS), 135n1
National Patient Safety Agency (NPSA), 93
neck stiffness, 3
needle stick injuries (NSI), 55
neutropenia, 48
NHS bodies, 137n37
NHS grades, 136n17
'no blame' culture, 92
non-English speaking patient, 37
noradrenaline, 4, 117
numb legs, 2

oblique phrases, 41
oesophageal cancer, 53
oesophageal varices, bleeding, 53

oesophagogastroduodenoscopy (OGD), 9
Offri, Danielle, 90, 91
one-to-one meetings, 107
openness, degree of, 73
optimism, 36, 37, 38
out-of-date knowledge, 116
out-patient clinic, 57–59
oxygen level, 4, 17, 87, 123
oxygen mask, 4, 35, 60
oxygen saturation, 5–6, 60

Page L, 137n32
pain
    abdominal, 51, 113, 125
    chest, 74, 107
    emotional, 33
    sensation of, 2
pain killers, 76
palliative care, 47, 128
pancreatic cancer, 47, 89
paralysis, 3, 19–22, 80, 98
paternalism, 73
Paterson, Ian, 83, 136n19
pejorative references, 133
pelvic bones, 3
penicillin, 68, 75, 93
peritonitis, 70, 112, 115, 135n4
personal accountability, 96, 98, 127
pessimism, 42
Peters D, 96, 137n30
Pink, Daniel, 96
platelet level, 7
pneumonia, 11, 16, 40–41, 73, 108, 128
pneumothoraces, 16
pneumothorax, 74, 122
polycystic liver disease, 39
positive end expiratory pressure (PEEP), 15
positive energy, 1
positive experiences, 1, 133
potential accountability, 92
potential disaster, 54
premature retirement, 81
'preparatory' conversation, 40
pride, 1, 5–8, 13, 56, 107
Procrustean couch, 10
professionalism, 33
professional 'stress', 100
protected disclosure, 119
proximal, 126, 127
psychogenic non-epileptic seizures (PNES), 60
psychological distress, 101
PTSD-type symptoms, 100
public service, working in, 134
pulmonary oedema, 4

Queen Elizabeth Hospital (QEH), 119
query aspiration, 19, 135–136n8

Reason J, 93, 137n28
reassurance, 10, 34, 35, 82, 96, 125, 131
rectal cancer, 23
renal failure, 19, 93
resilience, 51, 96, 97, 133
    burst, 79–83
    curve, 83–87
    distance, 55–65
    eyeroll, 94–101
    fear, 90–94
    guilt, 68–70
    judgement, 87–90
    poison, 76–78
    right, 51–53
    sorry, 70–76
    stick, 54–55
    sweat, 65–67
    try, 78–79
    wall, 53–54
respiratory distress, 19
responsibility, 15, 51, 93, 95, 104, 105, 110
resuscitation, 3, 17, 35, 41–42, 75, 138n42
retirement, premature, 81
retrospection, 125, 126
retrospectoscope, 90
'routine' conversation, 42
Royal College of Surgeons (RCS), 71

schistosomiasis, 23, 136n9
Scorsese, Martin, x
Scott SD, 136n14
second victim, 67, 99, 137n34
self-congratulation, 6
self-esteem, 2
Sellu, David, 112–116
senior house officer (SHO), 10, 12
seniority, 106, 133
sensation, loss of, 2
sensory change, 2
septicaemia, ix
septic shock, ix, 74, 117, 118
shared responsibility, 109, 110
Shem, Samuel, 136n11
sophistry, 9, 87
spinal cord tumour, 2
spinal muscular atrophy, 19, 45
spinal stimulator, 28
spontaneous bacterial peritonitis, 10
Starzl, Tom, 85
Stock B, 87, 137n22

stomach cancer, 20
stress, 1, 26, 55, 69
    everyday, 99
    professional, 100
stroke, 39, 80
strongyloides, 11–12
Stuff Happens (2004) (play), 66, 136n13
sub-optimalism, 100
'sub-optimal' decisions, 90
substandard medical care, 107
success, 1
supervisor, educational, 68, 75, 93, 98, 103, 110
surgery, 17, 27, 28, 31
    brain, 64
    cardiothoracic, 82, 85
    emergency, 80, 125
    heart, 82
    plastic surgery, 44
    vascular, 8
surgical cure, 47
swallowing problem, 8

Talbot, Simon, 98
tamponade, 16
This Is Going to Hurt (Adam Kay), 51
thyroid hormone, 1
training, 1, 11, 94
training encounter form, 111
transurethral resection of the prostate (TURP), 135n7
'trial and error', degree of, 85
turf, 44, 136n11
TURP patients, 17, 137n7

ulcer, 83–84
ultimate responsibility, 127
unconsciousness, 35, 137n36
urinary infection, ix, 11, 116

vascular surgery, 8
vasculitis, 12
venous thromboembolisms (VTE), 87–88
Verghese, Abraham, 34
vodka, 24, 27

Walter, Dan, 66–67
ward-appropriate, 43
Wilson JA, 137n20
wins, 1
With The End in Mind (2018), xii
Woodward, Theodore E., 135n2
words, 31, 33

Milton Keynes UK
Ingram Content Group UK Ltd.
UKHW031151141024
449569UK00024B/873